THE NAKED SURGEON

Samer Nashef, who qualified as a doctor at the University of Bristol in 1980, is a consultant cardiac surgeon at Papworth Hospital, Cambridge, and a world-leading expert on risk and quality in surgical care. He is the creator of EuroSCORE, which calculates the predicted risk of death from heart operations and is the most successful risk model in medicine; it is used worldwide and is credited with saving tens of thousands of lives. The author of more than 200 publications, Nashef's research has been widely cited, and he has been invited to lecture in more than 30 countries. He is a clinical tutor at the University of Cambridge, and is also a dedicated teacher and public communicator, having appeared in NHS Direct videos, at the Wellcome Trust foundation, and in Channel 4's *The Operation*. Outside the world of medicine, he is a regular compiler of cryptic crosswords for *The Guardian* and the *Financial Times* under a pseudonym.

To my mother
and
Neil Armstrong

(and to all the other patients who died after heart surgery)

THE
NAKED
SURGEON

the power and peril

of transparency in medicine

Samer Nashef

SCRIBE
Melbourne • London

Scribe Publications
18–20 Edward St, Brunswick, Victoria 3056, Australia
2 John St, Clerkenwell, London, WC1N 2ES, United Kingdom

First published by Scribe 2015
This edition published 2016

Typeset in Minion by the publishers

Printed and bound in the UK by CPI Group (UK) Ltd, Croydon CR0 4YY

Scribe Publications is committed to the sustainable use of natural resources
and the use of paper products made responsibly from those resources.

9781925106664 (Australian edition)
9781925228694 (UK edition)
9781925113808 (e-book)

CiP records for this title are available from the National Library of Australia
and the British Library

scribepublications.com.au
scribepublications.co.uk

Contents

Primum non nocere
(first, do no harm)

There are three kinds of doctor:
those who can count …
and those who can't.

Foreword

I had the pleasure of being a colleague of Samer Nashef after his appointment as a consultant at Papworth Hospital in 1992. It soon became apparent that we had added an unusually gifted and stimulating surgeon to our team. He already had a wide experience across the field of adult cardiac surgery, and was a fine technical surgeon and wise clinician. He also had the habit of questioning received wisdom, which encouraged us to look critically at procedures and see how these could be improved.

In due course, the latter propensity became a driving ambition to help cardiac surgeons to become more transparent about their results. This in turn led to creating the EuroSCORE model for predicting the outcome of heart operations, so that individual and national groups of surgeons could compare their results. The model became widely applied across Europe and beyond, and acted as an important stimulus for improving the results of cardiac surgery, thereby saving many lives.

Nashef's book gives interesting examples of his investigations into factors affecting outcomes, such as whether surgeons should operate immediately after a death on the table, and whether the risk-propensity of individual surgeons is measurable and can affect their results. He has a gift for making complex issues understandable, and presents the means by which patients can use mortality data to help them come to informed decisions about the risks and benefits of treatments offered them. At a more general level, he provides powerful arguments against some of the ill-conceived targets and rankings created by non-professionals that hospitals have been subjected to, and shows how these can mislead patients and demoralise doctors.

The Naked Surgeon is altogether a very stimulating read and one that will be of great interest to both patients and doctors. It should also receive the attention it deserves from health politicians, hospital managers, and health economists.

Sir Terence English, KBE, FRCS, FRCP
Past President of the Royal College of Surgeons of England

Prologue

As a medical student in 1977, I had a profound dislike of surgeons. They tended, I thought, to combine arrogance with a stunning ignorance of most aspects of medicine to which they could not take a knife. Many of my fellow students felt the same. While this was initially due to youthful prejudice on my part, over the course of my training I stumbled upon some disturbing facts about the practice of surgery that revealed my bias to have been based in truth.

In British medical schools in the '70s, students were attached to 'firms' for varying periods, usually of a few weeks. Firms were hospital sub-units made of a pair or a trio of senior doctors, or 'consultants', working in one specialty, such as general surgery, or general medicine, or general surgery with an interest in urology, and so forth. We medical students tagged along on the firm's ward rounds, sat in clinics, sometimes asked questions, and other times tried to answer them. Occasionally, we were directly taught at the bedside or in a corridor, if the opportunity arose and if the busy and harassed doctor we were trailing felt inclined to teach. In exchange for this 'medical education by osmosis', we were expected to help the junior doctors with 'clerking' duties (endless paperwork and form-filling), but our most crucial and useful task consisted of taking an impossibly large number of daily blood samples from patients. These were for the tests needed to make a

1

diagnosis and manage the patients' progress during their hospital stay. And so we went, from firm to firm, trying to learn, enjoying the hospital environment, and, vampire-like, taking countless blood samples.

My next firm was to be the professorial surgical firm, distinguished by being 'academic': in other words, some of its senior surgeons, in addition to being consultants, had university positions with titles such as 'lecturer' or 'professor'. These were somewhat more prestigious and grand surgeons who, in addition to operating on patients, were expected to be keen and dedicated teachers and researchers. During a two-month stint, students on this firm did all the usual clerking work and blood samples, but were also given an additional assignment. We were each allocated a topic to read about, and we were required, on the last Friday of our attachment to the firm, to give a short talk on the chosen topic to a small and select assembly consisting of the firm surgeons, professor, and lecturers, as well as our fellow students.

My assigned topic was 'emergency arterial surgery', which sounded pretty exotic. Not much surgery was done on arteries in those days, so such operations, and emergency ones to boot, promised to be an eye-opener.

I managed to find two examples of such surgery. The first was a 'femoral embolectomy', the removal of a blood clot from the main artery to the leg. This is what happens: A patient with a problematic heart gets a blood clot in it. As the heart beats, the clot becomes detached (in medical parlance, it becomes an 'embolus', or roving clot) and travels out of the heart and down the body until it gets stuck in the femoral artery, the large blood vessel that feeds the leg. The leg becomes cold, white, and painful, and, unless the clot is quickly removed by femoral embolectomy, the leg dies and drops off, or has to be amputated. Now that is drastic surgery, but it is quite tame when compared with the second example I found: repair of a ruptured 'abdominal aortic aneurysm' (or 'triple A').

The aorta is the biggest artery in the body, with the calibre of a large hosepipe. It comes out of the top of the heart, curves back like an old-fashioned walking stick, and descends through the chest towards the belly and the legs, giving branches along the way that feed every single part of the body. Sometimes, the wall of the aorta, as it passes through the belly, is weakened by age and disease. Under the relentless high pressure of the blood within it, it begins to stretch out into a balloon, or 'aneurysm'. Eventually, it suffers the inevitable fate of most balloons: it bursts. When this particular balloon bursts, the patient either dies suddenly or becomes very sick, in shock, with lots of blood and clots in the belly, and, unless an emergency operation is done immediately to replace the blown bit of aorta with a watertight plastic tube, death is certain.

I began my research by visiting the library to find out more about ruptured triple A: what causes it, who gets it, what its symptoms are, how it is fixed, and what percentage of patients survive. I quickly discovered that, despite treatment by emergency surgery, about half the patients died. It occurred to me that I might find some individual patient stories with which to enliven my talk, and to look at the experience with this operation locally. At the time, not much had been written about this rare condition, so, being rather ambitious, I resolved to study all cases of ruptured triple A treated in the hospital in the previous ten years.

It was a daunting task. In those days, there were no electronic clinical databases. All patient data were on paper in the medical records department, where old case notes were chaotically stacked high and wide in the vast, windowless, and musty basement of the hospital. There was an opaque card-filing system, which was poorly organised and not fully understood even by the clerk who presided over that shadowy underworld. This was going to be a tedious trawl. After spending every spare hour in that basement for more than a month, I eventually emerged with the case notes of 46 patients with ruptured triple A.

I summarised all the patient features, the findings at operation, and the outcomes of these operations. I then analysed the results with an eye to what determines a successful outcome: survival. I was taken aback to discover that all of my hypotheses for important factors in survival were simply wrong. I had assumed that unduly delayed diagnosis would lead to death. It didn't. I had guessed that unduly delayed treatment would lead to death. It didn't. I had thought that older and sicker patients, or those whose kidneys had shut down, were more likely to die. They weren't.

Two factors alone predicted the outcome. The first was how badly the patient was in shock on arrival at the hospital: those who arrived cold and clammy with a fast heart rate and a low blood pressure did badly, and those who were pink at the edges with good circulation and a normal blood pressure did well. The second factor was who did the operation. To my astonishment, the best results had been achieved by a pair of surgeons with a special interest in breast and thyroid surgery, and the worst results by the firm that actually specialised in arteries, which was — you guessed it — the very firm of surgeons to which I was attached. As for the causes of death, they were varied, but, on post-mortem examination, more than half were found to have had technical problems, such as bleeding from the stitch lines.

This was dynamite! How was it possible that the surgeons who should have been the best at this operation were actually the worst? What was going on?

Convinced that I was onto something big, I double-checked

my results and presented them in a brief written report. I also summarised the findings on some overhead transparency sheets, the last of which listed all the surgeons by name against their success rates. That night, I went to the pub in a celebratory mood. At the very least, I had an excellent talk to give. At best, there would be a scientific paper of enormous interest to surgeons: not at all bad for a third-year medical student.

The last Friday of the attachment finally arrived. It was a beautiful sunny day when we all trooped into the small lecture theatre clutching our overhead transparencies. My talk was at the end of the programme, so I waited and listened politely, albeit with a little impatience, while my fellow students delivered their reports and answered questions from the consultants. At long last, it was my turn. I rose to the podium, placed my first transparency on the overhead projector, and began talking. The audience appeared moderately interested as I reported on patients, told their stories, quoted the numbers, and explained my analysis. The level of attention rose perceptibly as I started talking about outcomes and factors associated with survival. Towards the end of the talk, I began to speak about the link between surgeons and outcomes, when a palpable coldness permeated the atmosphere in the room. I placed my last transparency on the overhead projector.

On the left-hand side of the projected transparency was a column of survival rates, in descending order, from around 70 per cent to around 25 per cent. On the right-hand side was a list of surgeons' names, covered with a blank sheet of paper. I then asked the audience if they wanted to see the names. There was total and absolute silence. Nobody coughed, shifted, or even audibly breathed.

The talk was not going well.

After what seemed an interminably long time, a senior lecturer (who later went on to become a famous professor of surgery) looked around him and said: 'Well, I'm not particularly interested. Is anyone?' The few mumbled grunts and coughs that followed clearly indicated that nobody else was particularly interested either. As I gathered my bits of paper, the audience filed out of the room. There was to be no feedback, no praise, and certainly no paper to publish. When the grades for that attachment were delivered, I was awarded a C minus — a borderline pass — with a bonus feature: a personalised handwritten addendum describing this particular student as 'arrogant and unaware of his own deficiencies'.

Two years later, we were approaching the end of medical school, and the time had come to apply for jobs as house officers — the most junior doctors in a hospital. All new graduates had to work for six months as a house officer in a surgical specialty and another six months in a medical specialty before they were given full registration with the General Medical Council and let loose on patients. I had no difficulty in securing a good house job in a medical specialty at my own teaching hospital, but, when it came to the surgical house job, it was a different story. Frustratingly, most of my applications to posts in the region were rejected even before the interview stage. After a prolonged and anxious wait, I was relieved to be asked to attend an interview for the post of house officer to a consultant surgeon in a district general hospital some 40 miles away from my medical school. I dug out my regulation charcoal pinstripe suit, sober tie, and worn but serviceable black shoes, and arrived at the interview with three other candidates.

I walked into the office and saw the surgeon, an elegant, slim, and smartly dressed young consultant whom I recognised immediately: he had been a senior trainee surgeon in the academic surgical firm two years previously.

'Oh, it's you', he said, as he looked up from his papers and saw me.

'I'm afraid it is', I said, trying to sound cheerful.

'Terrible business, that was, terrible business ...' he added, as he escorted me back to the office door. 'Anyway, if it makes you feel any better, I have kept a copy of your study, and have read it and referred to it more than once. Next candidate, please.'

The interview was over. It suddenly dawned on me that, as a result of my medical student project, I was being blacklisted (either officially or unofficially) for surgical jobs in the region. I had crashed headlong into surgeons' arrogant refusal to examine the results of their operations.

After that, I hated surgeons.

Out of the Dark Ages

It is remarkable to think that, until a couple of hundred years ago, medicine and its myriad forms of treatment were administered to patients almost as an act of faith. Much of early medicine had no basis in science or fact, and only in modern times have our treatments been supported by at least some hard evidence that they actually work. Once we have discovered effective treatments, an obvious next step would be to find out how well they are administered. Yet this is a question that had not even begun to be asked until the last couple of decades or so, when the scrutiny of medical outcomes began in earnest.

Today, most medical treatment is supported by scientific evidence, and most doctors claim to practise medicine that is 'evidence-based'. We are therefore abundantly justified in beginning to ask the question I posed to my peers as a medical student: how well do those who treat us actually treat us?

I am now a heart surgeon, and proud of the fact. I know that I do many patients a lot of good (and a very few untold harm), but the net effect of my interventions, like that of most of my colleagues, is overwhelmingly positive. That said, I would not have been proud to be a surgeon, or indeed any kind of medical doctor, a hundred years or more ago. Many, if not most, of the medical treatments dished out with tremendous authority and style by my ancient predecessors to long-suffering patients over the centuries were not only useless, but actually downright harmful.

I am referring here not to quack doctors, 'alternative medicine' practitioners, homeopaths, and faith healers, but to properly qualified physicians who had sworn the Hippocratic Oath. These highly educated 'doctors' treated syphilis with mercury, a seriously toxic metal that did nothing to alleviate the disease. They managed a multitude of conditions with entirely useless bloodletting and leeches, and another multitude with enforced bed-rest cures and ludicrously long confinements to sanatoria. They performed unnecessary circumcisions, bowel removals, and many other dubious operations, causing horrific and often fatal infections by operating in filthy theatres with no sterility, asepsis, or even basic hygiene. To make matters worse, they usually carried out this carnage with supreme self-confidence. The idea that one should have some kind of proof of effectiveness before administering a treatment to a patient would have been alien to them.

In the past century, we have moved from this barely disguised witchcraft to therapies that actually work, allowing us more often than not to give the correct treatment for a particular condition. And, in the past two decades, we have seen the advent of a second revolution in healthcare: the long-overdue introduction of the concept of quality control in medicine. We have just started to ensure that, having chosen the correct treatment, it is delivered safely and well.

In this book, I explore how the concept of quality measurement came to be an essential part of medical and surgical practice. In the timeline of thousands of years of medical practice, good and bad, the concept was born only yesterday. For many years, the profession simply did not want to know about measures of quality. As I discovered to my cost a mere three decades ago, even asking the question about the quality of healthcare delivery was sufficient to produce ostracism.*

Ironically, these events took place at the same hospital where, a few years later, a failure of quality control exploded into a scandal that brought about a sea change in medical practice and attitudes. What's more, the scandal involved the specialty in which I eventually qualified: heart surgery.

The first intimations that things were not as they should be in the Bristol paediatric heart surgery came on 8 May 1992, when the British satirical magazine *Private Eye* first drew attention to the high mortality of heart surgery in children at the Bristol Royal Infirmary. The professional who, at great risk to himself and his medical career, helped expose the scandal at Bristol was Dr Steve Bolsin. When he was appointed as a consultant anaesthetist in Bristol in 1988, he saw a charming city in an idyllic setting in which he and his wife, Maggie, would raise their family. He never expected Bristol, as he put it, to become the graveyard of his dreams at the same time as it became the graveyard of many children who could have survived if they had been operated on elsewhere.

Soon after starting to work in the department of paediatric

---

* In the grand scheme of things, my blacklisting for surgical jobs was a fairly mild form of victimisation. I merely stopped looking for training posts in the region surrounding my teaching hospital and applied for two posts in other cities, much further away. I was immediately offered them both, and the pleasant dilemma was which one to choose.

heart surgery in Bristol, Bolsin noticed that the operations were taking an inordinately long time and that the survival rate was not as good as he thought it should be. A few months later, an audit meeting of the paediatric cardiac surgical specialists confirmed his suspicions that the death rates in Bristol were abnormally high. These were not small differences: death rates were many times greater in Bristol than should be expected, and that was true for even some standard, relatively simple heart operations. In the case of some of the more intricate, newly developed operations, the death rate was absolutely appalling.

He also made another shocking discovery: it soon became apparent to him that the poor standards and results were something of an open secret. Many people 'in the know' fully realised that Bristol was endangering children's lives in its heart surgery programme, yet most of them refrained from blowing the whistle and took no remedial action. The professionals in the field talked about it, and, in some cases, physicians took active steps to avoid sending their own patients to Bristol. For the cities of Cardiff and Plymouth, Bristol was geographically the closest paediatric heart unit, yet the children's heart specialists there were sending their patients to Southampton, a heart unit much further away. In fact, the children from Wales and their families would have to drive past Bristol to reach Southampton for surgery.

Despite all this, little was done to address the problem in Bristol for several years, and it was only through the courage of Bolsin that the situation ultimately came to a head. After personally investigating and reviewing the data, he expressed his concerns several times within the department, and beyond the department to the hospital management structure. On all occasions, he was given the brush-off, and, on some occasions, he was threatened.

Finally, he blew the whistle.*

These disclosures made medical history. They led to a massive healthcare scandal and a public inquiry specifically and poignantly centred on the poor results achieved by paediatric heart surgeons. The scale of the inquiry was unprecedented. The families of children with heart defects treated in Bristol were invited to give evidence. In addition, the inquiry heard from Bristol doctors, healthcare workers, and managers. Medical experts from other centres and representatives of specialist organisations and colleges from around the nation were also called in as witnesses. The total cost was estimated at around £15 million. The report was published in 2001. It revealed that, between 1984 and 1995, the lives of as many as 171 children could have been spared if they had been operated on anywhere other than Bristol. The report also made 198 recommendations dealing with the need for robust monitoring of outcomes, transparency of medical-outcome data, and a host of other issues related to the quality of care. Along with the public outcry at the scandal, these recommendations contributed to the transformation of the culture that had prevailed in medicine at the time. The medical profession had been served with a wake-up call. From then on, it became unacceptable to treat patients with no regard to the standard of clinical outcomes. The pernicious combination of secrecy, complacency, and arrogance that had afflicted much of the medical establishment in the past was at last under effective assault. The concept of quality measurement in medicine had arrived.

Besides the Bristol scandal, there are several other reasons why heart surgery has driven advances in this field. For a start, the

---

* Bolsin found it impossible to continue living and working in Bristol, and left the country for Australia. His account of the events leading to the scandal appears in Appendix A.

specialty involves a relatively limited number of operations, with coronary bypass and valve operations accounting for most of our work. It also has a performance outcome that is easily measurable and difficult to argue with: survival (or death, depending on your outlook). What's more, the specialty has been measuring these outcomes since its inception — as a relatively young specialty, it could only develop by demonstrating outcomes good enough to justify its invasive approach, which originally involved great risk relative to conventional drug treatment. Finally, heart surgery has well-developed risk models that allow us to predict the likely outcome of treatment. By comparing the predicted outcome with the actual outcome, we have a pretty good idea how well (or badly) we are doing.

What is amazing about heart surgery is not that it exists and works, but that it took so long to appear. After all, the heart is a pump, pure and simple. When something goes wrong with a pump, it is a plumbing problem, needing plumbing solutions. How else do you fix a blockage in a pipe, or a leaky valve? Yet, for more than 2000 years, the heart was exclusively the domain of the physician, not the surgeon, and woe betide the surgeon who dared touch it. The taboo on operating on the heart was so strong that Theodor Billroth, one of the great founding fathers of modern surgery, stated in 1889 that 'a surgeon who tries to suture a heart wound deserves to lose the esteem of his colleagues'.

There were two main reasons why the heart could not be tackled surgically. The first actually had to do with the lungs. These are the sponge-like organs that exchange gases with the air. They inflate and deflate a dozen times a minute to bring in oxygen and get rid of carbon dioxide. The problem is that the lungs do not do this by themselves, because they are entirely passive structures. The lungs inflate and deflate only by following the chest wall around them as it expands and contracts with the muscles of breathing. There is a sealed vacuum between the lungs and the chest wall, so that the lungs must follow the movements of the chest wall with every breath. Opening the chest to operate on anything inside it breaks that seal and lets air into the cavity. The lungs then fall away from the chest wall, and breathing stops immediately. At first, our intrepid pioneering heart surgeon would have been pleased to see this: there is suddenly a lot of room in the chest, and the heart can be easily reached. Sadly, his joy would have been short-lived, because the patient would have died a few minutes later from lack of oxygen. This was the fate of patients in whom chest surgery was attempted until the second half of the 19th century, when the endotracheal tube was invented. By inserting this tube into the windpipe (trachea), air or oxygen could be actively blown into the lungs. This made a lot of anaesthesia safer and more controlled. It also made major open-chest operations possible for the first time.

The second reason was the heart itself. This little muscle, about the size of your fist, pumps five litres of blood every minute to deliver oxygen and nourishment to the entire body. In fact, the average adult only has about five litres of blood in total, so your entire lifeblood goes full circle around your whole body every single minute of your life. If the heart stops, death follows almost immediately, as the body cannot live without a blood supply. Different parts of the body, however, are not equally sensitive to the loss of their blood supply for a short while. Your leg will probably recover if its blood supply is cut for half an hour, but your brain most certainly will not normally survive more than a few minutes without blood and oxygen.

Operating on the heart involves touching it, twisting it, pressing on it, and sometimes turning it upside down. All of these manoeuvres interfere with the pumping action, so any heart operation that disrupted the pumping action of the heart for more than a few minutes was likely to cause brain damage or death. Thus, the only operations that could be done on the heart were ultra-short ones: a few minutes to cobble up a hole and hope for the best marked the limit of what heart surgeons could do. This unhappy state of affairs remained until the middle of the 20th century, when the heart–lung machine was invented: a contraption that took over the job of the heart and lungs, keeping the patient alive while surgeons fiddled with the heart. After the first successful use of the machine, in 1953 by John Gibbon in Philadelphia, USA, everything changed: this marvellous invention opened the door wide and ushered in the new specialty of cardiac surgery.

The invention of the heart–lung machine was to heart surgery as the starter pistol is to an Olympic sprint runner. The specialty took off and ran with breathtaking, almost indecent, speed, so that, by the 1960s, heart surgery was no longer considered crazy. More and more patients were being saved, more sophisticated and complex operations were being invented, and the results were looking better and better. The specialty was transformed from a very limited last-ditch intervention in otherwise hopeless cases to a routine part of modern medicine's armamentarium. Not surprisingly, units specialising in heart surgery mushroomed in major hospitals in many countries fortunate enough to have access to the resources for high-tech (and expensive) healthcare.

In the early 1980s, when I was working as a medical house officer at the Bristol Royal Infirmary, the heart surgery unit was a truly intimidating place. Mere medical house officers like me were the lowest of the low in the pecking order of hospital medicine, and were probably not welcomed there. Even if we had been welcomed, we were profoundly ignorant of what went on behind the door with the forbidding sign 'Cardiac intensive care unit — do not enter'. Heart surgery formed no part of our undergraduate medical curriculum because it was considered too specialised and newfangled for mere student doctors. Nevertheless, whenever my bosses, the cardiology consultant physicians, decided that one of our patients could perhaps benefit from having a heart operation, it was my duty as a house officer and general gofer to deliver the carefully written referral note to one of the cardiac surgeons.

Even in my complete ignorance of cardiac surgery and utter obliviousness of its outcomes, I could not help noticing that there was a tendency to insist on referral to a particular surgeon in certain cases. Perhaps these were difficult cases, or patients that the cardiologist cared deeply about, but occasionally I would be given this instruction: 'Make sure this referral goes to Mr Wisheart and nobody else. We want this one to live.'

Several years later, Mr Wisheart, a senior surgeon, found himself at the centre of the Bristol heart scandal. He was struck off the medical register for, among other reasons, having too *high* a death rate for certain operations. His subjective reputation among the local cardiologists was clearly not borne out by the hard data. The whole episode graphically illustrates the dangers inherent in not knowing if the quality of clinical outcomes is failing to reach acceptable standards, and in not acting when that knowledge becomes available. Much has changed for the better since then. Bristol is now considered to be a centre of excellence, and other heart surgery units have also improved massively as a result of the lessons learned from Bristol.

Together with quality measurement, the concept of clinical governance was introduced as a result of the Bristol event, and is now accepted as essential for the conduct of medical care. Clinical governance places the responsibility of clinical outcomes directly

2

The Benchmark Operation

There is a major difference between the public perception of surgeons (doctors who treat mainly by cutting patients) and physicians (doctors who treat mainly by prescribing drugs). When a physician treats a patient, and the patient dies, then it is commonly seen as the patient's fault: he or she 'failed to respond' to the treatment. This platitude becomes harder to swallow if the treatment is an elective operation: when a healthy patient walks into a hospital, has an operation, and then dies, it is much easier to think that the surgeon was at fault. After all, the temporal, if not causal, relationship between the operation and the outcome speaks with a resonant eloquence that is impossible to ignore. Nowhere is this relationship in sharper focus than in heart surgery: a heart operation that goes wrong leads more directly and more rapidly to death than, say, an orthopaedic or bowel operation.

One of the simplest clinical outcomes to measure is the death rate of an operation. When 100 patients have an operation and five die as a result, we say the mortality of the operation is 5 per cent. This simple percentage is a crude yet crucial measure of an operation's success rate, and its importance was recognised as far back as the 1960s by Michael Crichton.

Crichton, who died in 2008 at the age of only 66, was a prolific American writer of novels, film scripts, and television series (including *Jurassic Park* and *ER*). He developed a keen interest in writing at a young age, but moved from studying literature to medicine while at Harvard Medical School. One of his early novels, *A Case of Need*, begins with the intriguing statement 'All heart surgeons are bastards'. A page later, he describes one particular (fictional) heart surgeon in the following terms:

> Because Frank Conway was good, because he was an eight-percenter, a man with lucky hands, a man with the touch, everyone put up with his temper tantrums, his moments of anger and destructiveness.

Many anaesthetists, operating room nurses, and trainee surgeons will sympathise with this profile, and perhaps recognise some of their own heart surgeons in this damning depiction, but much more important than the vivid description of surgical tantrums is the term 'eight-percenter'. This is the surgeon's mortality rate: the proportion of patients who die under the knife, so to speak, or soon after the operation.

Fortunately, we have come a long way from the days when 8 per cent mortality in heart surgery was considered evidence of excellence. Nowadays, the death rate after heart surgery in many great hospitals around the world is approximately 2 per cent, or even lower, but what is truly interesting about this passage in Michael Crichton's book is not the percentage. It is this: even as far back as the 1960s, and in the eyes of a populist writer of mass-market medical fiction, albeit one studying medicine at one of the top medical schools in the world, the measurement of the quality of a heart surgeon's work was well and truly established in people's minds as the percentage mortality. This, rudimentary and crude as it may be, was probably the first sign of quality control and performance measurement in medicine.

On the face of it, the death rate after a particular type of operation is a straightforward measure of how good the operator and the hospital are. It is one definition of success that is crucial for at least two reasons. First, it is absolute: after an operation, the patient is either dead or alive.* Second, the patient needs to be alive to enjoy the benefits of whatever was done, so the patient will care more about survival than about other possible benefits, such as quality of life and symptom relief, which, important though they are, do not count for much if one is dead.

In heart surgery, the benchmark procedure (or 'index procedure') for measuring the quality of medical care is an operation used to treat angina. Having angina is bad news. For a start, it feels awful. It does not hurt in the same way that a paper cut or a hammer blow to your thumb does, but it is truly unpleasant. Angina is a perception of tightness or pressure across the chest, and usually comes on with physical exertion. Patients may describe it as a sensation of heaviness, a dead weight, or a vice-like grip. It does not score high on the pain severity scale, but it is often associated with a feeling of impending doom that, at the very least, makes you want to stop or slow down your physical exertions until it abates. Angina is heartache, literally.

More importantly, having angina means your coronary arteries are narrowed, and that is even worse news. A coronary artery becomes narrowed when its wall is furred up with cholesterol. The resulting formation is called a 'plaque'. A plaque can rupture, and,

---

* Though even such a simple outcome can, in practice, be difficult to define and a subject of controversy. This is addressed in Chapter Four.

when that happens, the cholesterol and other coarse muck within it become exposed to the blood flowing within the artery. The blood then sticks to the disrupted plaque and forms a clot, and the narrowed coronary artery closes completely. The bit of heart muscle that the coronary artery supplies begins to die, and this is called a heart attack. As everyone knows, heart attacks kill people. Having angina means that the sufferer, in addition to the pain that is angina, is at a higher risk of having a heart attack.

Fortunately, angina can now be cured (and the risk of heart attack dramatically reduced) by the most commonly performed heart operation ever: coronary artery bypass grafting, or CABG for short. In this operation, veins or arteries are taken from various body parts and used to bypass blockages or narrowings in the coronary arteries, those fine, fiddly, yet fiendishly important vital suppliers to the heart muscle itself. The operation is done to relieve the heartache that is angina and to help prevent heart attacks. The layperson calls this operation a bypass, or a double, triple, or quadruple bypass, depending on the number of coronary arteries that are treated and how much the patient wants to impress the select few who are remotely interested in someone else's tales of medical adventure. Heart surgeons and cardiologists often just call it a 'cabbage', a corruption of the acronym CABG. Politically correct hospital managers really do not like the use of the term 'cabbage', especially when there are patients or relatives within earshot. They prefer to call it 'See a Bee Gee' (singing 'Stayin' Alive', perhaps?).

I hope your coronary arteries are as clean and unobstructed as the day you were born, but, perish the thought, let us assume they are not. Perhaps years of smoking, obesity, and high blood pressure have taken their toll, or you have led a clean and healthy life but were cursed by a family genetic predisposition to plaque formation in the arteries. Whatever the cause, you now have angina that no number of tablets can relieve, a family history littered with early deaths from heart attacks, and coronary arteries full of blockages and narrowings. In short, you have been advised to have a CABG.

You have decided to go ahead, and your next decision is to choose between surgeon A and surgeon B. Both are nice people, friendly, men, of a similar age, have an excellent bedside manner, and work in the same hospital. In fact, you find it difficult to distinguish between them in most respects, but then you learn their mortality data: surgeon A has a CABG mortality of 1.25 per cent, and surgeon B has a CABG mortality of 2.08 per cent — nearly double that of surgeon A. Which surgeon would you choose? Surgeon A, of course! This, as some would say, is a no-brainer.

But is it? You could, in fact, be making a very big mistake.

Consider the situation in more detail. You are a prospective patient contemplating having a CABG at St Elsewhere's General Infirmary. You do your homework and obtain information about the hospital, its location and services, the quality of its food, its policy on visiting hours, and, perhaps most important of all, the ease and cost of parking your car there. You also, wisely, ask for data on the various heart surgeons and their CABG results. The hospital obliges willingly, as it has a policy of openness and transparency coupled with pride in the results. The information is provided to you by the hospital's audit department. The data have been validated by a specialist society and published on the web for all to see. It simply states that, for CABG, the benchmark operation for measuring performance, the results are as follows:

CABG mortality at St Elsewhere's General Infirmary	
Surgeon A	1.25%
Surgeon B	2.08%

On the face of it, the decision is indeed a no-brainer, but I first need to tell you a few things about surgeons A and B that do not appear in the figures. Surgeon B is an ordinary bloke, with a Type B personality. He drives an ageing Saab, is a little obsessive about safety, hates taking risks, and practises medicine on the basis of scientific evidence. Surgeon A, however, has a Type A personality. He drives a Ferrari, cuts corners in the operating theatre as on the road, likes to take risks in his own life and with the lives of his patients, and believes that evidence-based medicine is like painting by numbers — all right for pedestrian artists, but not for him, the self-styled Leonardo da Vinci of the art of surgery. Furthermore, he is getting a little bored with CABG as a blandly predictable, bread-and-butter operation, and wants to explore new ways of treating his patients.

In fact, most medicine as practised nowadays is (or at least should be) evidence-based. There is so much medical research around that a doctor should be armed with the facts and figures before deciding to use this or that type of treatment. The opposite of evidence-based medicine is sometimes practised by stubborn yet famous high-profile doctors. I call it eminence-based medicine, and it is defined as 'persisting in making the same mistake over and over again, but with ever-increasing conviction'. This is, of course, insane.

So we now have a mental picture of surgeon B as a solid citizen and surgeon A as a cavalier risk-taker. But, I hear you say, despite all that, surgeon A's CABG mortality is definitely lower, and that is surely a good thing. In fact, it is not.

To understand why, we need some additional information about the two surgeons and their CABG practice. Last year, two lots of 100 identically matched CABG patients were referred for surgery, 100 to each of the two surgeons. This is how the patients are in each of these two identical groups:

- All 100 have triple-vessel coronary artery disease and need a triple CABG.
- Eighty have strong hearts and are low-risk patients.
- Sixteen have weak hearts due to damage from a previous heart attack, with a stable, old scar on the heart, and are medium-risk patients.
- Four have weak hearts due to damage from a previous heart attack, and the scar on the heart has ballooned into an aneurysm, which is slowly expanding. They are high-risk patients.

Both surgeons do exactly the same for the 80 low-risk patients: they perform a triple CABG. The mortality in this group is expected to be low. Seventy-nine of the 80 patients sail through the operation without a hitch. One unfortunate patient dies as a result of the operation.

Both surgeons do exactly the same for the four high-risk patients: they carry out a triple CABG and cut out the aneurysm. This is a dangerous surgery, and, not surprisingly, one patient out of the four dies as a result, and the other three do well.

In the medium-risk group of 16 patients, surgeon B does a triple CABG, which is all they needed. One dies and 15 survive, as can be expected. Surgeon A, however, gets excited about the scar on the heart. He imagines it to be an aneurysm. He is getting bored with just doing CABG and wants some variety in his professional life. He fancies a challenge and happens to be feeling somewhat overconfident at the time. He decides to cut out the scar, call this additional procedure an aneurysmectomy, and then reshape the heart to make it work better. Of course, he has no scientific proof for any of this, but who needs proof when one is a surgical superstar? So he proceeds, despite the total lack of evidence that this will do any good, and despite the fact that this will unnecessarily complicate the surgery. In this group, surgeon A has three deaths: the one that was expected, plus two more due to the bleeding and heart-rhythm problems that arose directly as a result of the unnecessary cutting of the heart to remove an 'aneurysm' that wasn't really there.

Each of the two surgeons has now completed the 100 operations. Surgeon B has three deaths, and surgeon A has five. They submit their results to the auditors, and this is what is published:

- Simple operation (the benchmark procedure): CABG on its own
- Surgeon B: two deaths out of 96 =   2.08 per cent
- Surgeon A: one death out of 80 =   1.25 per cent
- Surgeon A wins!

- Complex operation: CABG plus aneurysmectomy
- Surgeon B: one death out of 4 =   25 per cent
- Surgeon A: four deaths out of 20 =   20 per cent
- Surgeon A wins again!

'But', you may well object, 'that is completely crazy; figures for death cannot possibly be that misleading!' Most of the time you would be right, but not always.

The above example shows one rather extreme consequence of

something I shall call the 'category shift', and it is a phenomenon that comes into play especially when the wrong outcome measure is used. Earlier, Michael Crichton, like so many others, evaluated heart surgeons by their mortality: what percentage of their patients died as a result of surgery. Later, many specialist organisations, professional bodies, hospital auditors, and media health correspondents became interested in 'procedural mortality'; in other words, the death rate of a particular type of operation. More often than not, the operation first chosen for measurement is the one carried out most commonly. In heart surgery, that operation is CABG. This is now our benchmark, or index, procedure. For many years and in many institutions around the world, CABG mortality was the only outcome measure used in cardiac surgery and, indeed, in healthcare as a whole. In 1992, the state of New York was the first official administration to measure this outcome in its many hospitals and make the results available to the general public. The impact that this had on New York surgeons was substantial, and much of it was negative.

Imagine an average New York State surgeon in 1992. He* has been bumbling along, doing the best for his patients, and achieving acceptable results for the early '90s with a CABG mortality of 4 per cent, when a newspaper, out of the blue, publishes a league table for CABG mortality in which he is ranked alongside all the other surgeons in the state. We have to remember that his practice (and his income, sports car, and second home in Florida) all depend on his being referred patients on whom to operate. The publication of outcomes means that patients, who, after all, have a choice in the matter, are likely to seek the surgeon with a low or even the lowest

---

* Even today, the overwhelming majority of heart surgeons are male, but this is slowly changing.

mortality. With half an eye on next year's figures, our surgeon is in the middle of performing a CABG on a frail, elderly woman with many medical problems. The operation is not going at all well. It is technically difficult, the arteries are heavily diseased and challenging to suture, the heart is weak with a scar from a previous heart attack, and there is a lot of bleeding: in short, this patient looks like she might not make it. Like many American surgeons, this surgeon only does about 50 CABGs per year. If she dies, his mortality jumps from 4 per cent to 6 per cent, now well above the average. On the other hand, if he decides to tackle that scar, she is no longer a CABG case, but a CABG and something else, and therefore no longer an index procedure. The patient shifts into another category.

'Now that you mention it,' he says to his assistant, 'that scar looks more and more like an aneurysm to me …'

It is obviously difficult to track with any certainty how often this sort of behaviour happens, but there are reports that such 'gaming' has been observed and is in fact commonplace in the US (Shahian 2001). Patients have had 'aneurysm' repair when there wasn't one, tricuspid valve repair when it wasn't needed, and other ingenious additions of unnecessary manoeuvres to shift them out of the index-procedure category. I have tried to gauge the prevalence of such behaviour in the United Kingdom by conducting an anonymous online survey of all heart surgeons. The question I asked my fellow surgeons, and their responses, are outlined below:

> It is possible for a cardiac surgeon to modify the appearance of surgeon-specific outcomes by using 'category shift'. For example, in a CABG, adding a few stitches to the left ventricle and calling the operation CABG and LV aneurysm, or a couple of stitches

to the tricuspid valve to add tricuspid valve repair, or excising a sliver of aorta in an AVR to call it AVR and aortoplasty, or ascending aortic repair. There are other examples. The net result is that an operation is shifted from a lower risk category to a higher risk category. Have you ever done this?

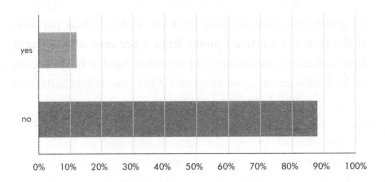

Are you aware of other surgeons doing this?

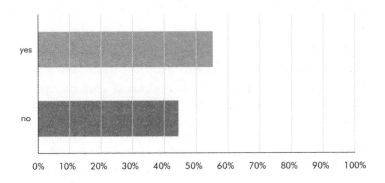

Of the 115 surgeons who responded, 12 (or just over 10 per cent) admitted to having practised category shift themselves, and more than half (55 per cent) stated that they were aware of other surgeons doing so.

The above findings illustrate the possible unpleasant consequences of a simple, well-meaning attempt at measuring the quality of a specialty service. The specialty is heart surgery, and the index procedure reasonably chosen to measure its quality is CABG, but the result of the exercise is a combination of damage to patients and unintentional muddying of the waters in the data pool. The problem with setting targets, as many health departments and ministers have discovered to their detriment and to that of their patients, is that, if you set the wrong target, you run the risk of distorting clinical decisions, with unexpected and sometimes damaging consequences. In fact, even if, with the best of intentions, you set the right target, but with insufficient consideration to the methods of measurement or to the human reaction to your plan, the law of unintended consequences may have some nasty surprises for you. The road to hell, as they say, is paved with good intentions.

In medicine, as in every field of human endeavour, we can choose what we want to measure. Sir Bruce Keogh, one-time cardiac surgeon and later medical director of the UK's National Health Service, used to ask this perceptive and thought-provoking question at meetings: 'Do we make what's important measurable, or what's measurable important?' It is a crucial question, for the simple reason that it is so tempting, when faced with something that is easy to measure, to fall into the trap of making that something important just because we can measure it easily. It is much more difficult to look at what actually matters to us, and to find a way of measuring it. This is a vital concept that should be drilled into all politicians and managers in charge of healthcare.

Our hypothetical New York surgeon replicated the behaviour

of surgeon A in producing category shift. Surgeon A did it out of ignorance and bloody-mindedness, and the New York surgeon did it semiconsciously with an eye on the league tables. Both of these instances are rather extreme representations of what can happen when the wrong targets are set, but there are even greater pitfalls than category shift in interpreting medical outcomes.

3

How Not to Lie with Statistics

Category shift is only one example where setting the wrong targets can lead to unwanted consequences that are bad for the patients, but at least it can be neutralised by setting intelligent targets and by truthful and wholesome reporting of outcomes. Let us assume that this happy state of affairs now prevails, and that our data have not been distorted by category shift or other misrepresentations. Can we now use mortality data to find out which surgeon or which hospital is the better one?

When surgeon X has a higher mortality rate than surgeon Y, there are three possible reasons: (1) the difference is due to chance alone; (2) the difference is due to different case mixes (surgeon X operates on many high-risk patients, say, and surgeon Y runs a mile when one comes along); or (3) surgeon Y is better. Before we can safely conclude that reason 3 is right, we must eliminate any possibility of reason 1 and reason 2.

Ensuring that the difference is not due to chance alone is actually remarkably easy to do, and has been one of the essential features of interpreting medical and other scientific research. The interpretation relies on basic statistics.

Imagine that you have a headache and you stumble upon a snake-oil salesman. He is flogging his snake oil as a treatment for headache. He confidently (and truthfully) asserts that, in his experience, 100 per cent of those who took the snake oil had their headache cured in an hour, whereas 100 per cent of those who didn't buy the snake oil still had a sore head after an hour. You might be suitably impressed, but you shouldn't be, or at least not yet. Before coming to any conclusions, you really, really must find out how many people with a headache took the snake oil and how many did not. You ask the snake-oil salesman, who replies (also truthfully) that only two people ever approached him with a headache. One took the oil and lost the headache, the other did not take the oil and the headache persisted. Does the snake oil work? Maybe it does and maybe it doesn't, but his earlier assertions are certainly no evidence for the efficacy of the medicine. Concluding that the snake oil works on the basis of this pathetic, two-patient, non-randomised clinical trial is exactly the same as stepping out of a cafe, meeting a six-foot-tall woman followed by a five-foot-11-inch-tall man, and concluding that women are taller than men. You cannot make such conclusions on the basis of so few observations. If, on the other hand, you measured the height of 10,000 women and 10,000 men at random in your town, and found that, on average, the women were six feet tall and the men only five feet, you would almost certainly be right in concluding that women are taller than men.

Statisticians are strange people in many ways. They tend to dissect data to death before telling us what the data mean, and one thing they never, ever do is jump to conclusions. In fact, there is an old joke about a journalist, a scientist, and a statistician on a train going through Scotland. They look out of the carriage window and see a black sheep on the hillside. The journalist exclaims: 'Wow, guys, look at that! Sheep are black in Scotland!' The scientist interjects: 'No, that's not strictly true. There are *some* sheep in Scotland that are black.' The statistician thinks for a long while, and finally says: 'I think we can safely conclude that, in Scotland, there appears to be at least one sheep, at least one side of which appears to be black.'

There is something absolutely fundamental to intelligent statistics, and it is this: the size of the sample. When we have data on a sample taken from a population, we need to know the size of the sample before jumping to any conclusions about that particular population. If we want to compare a feature between two populations, say for example the prevalence of blue eyes, then we might take a random sample of 100 people from population A and another 100 people from population B, and we count the number of people with blue eyes. Say we have 20 people with blue eyes in sample A and 21 in sample B. Does that mean that there are more blue-eyed people in population B? Probably not, as it seems highly likely that such a small difference may be simply due to chance. This means that a second important feature, once we have ascertained that the sample itself is of a decent size, is the size of any measured difference. Essentially, what we observe in the size of the samples and the size of the difference between them will determine, with appropriate statistical tests, how sure we can be that there is a real difference between the populations from which the samples were taken. There are, of course, other statistical measures, but the size of the sample and the size of the difference are sine qua non. No conclusion can be drawn without knowing them. An isolated observation obtained from looking at one lone sheep on the hillside tells you next to nothing about the nation's ovine population or its colouring characteristics.

There are pretty basic statistical tools that allow you to

determine the likelihood that a difference that is found is due purely to chance, and these tools usually express their results as a 'p-value'. The p-value is the probability that an observed difference is due to chance. If the p-value is 1, that means the difference is definitely due to chance. If it is 0.1, it means that there is a 10 per cent likelihood that the difference is due to chance. If it is 0.01, there is only a 1 per cent likelihood that the difference is due to chance. In medicine, as in many other scientific fields, the cut-off point has been arbitrarily set at 0.05: that means, if the likelihood of the difference being due to chance alone is less than 5 per cent, we conclude that the difference is real, or 'significant'. Anything more than 5 per cent, and the difference is non-significant: in other words, it doesn't cut the mustard. In a way, this is similar to the concept of the burden of proof in the practice of law. In a criminal court, the jury can only find the defendant guilty if it considers the case proven 'beyond reasonable doubt'. In a civil court, the decision can be made on 'the balance of probabilities'. In medical statistics, we make it easy: we actually measure the 'doubt'. More than 5 per cent: not guilty. Less than 5 per cent: guilty as charged.*

The story of the snake-oil salesman is not as far-fetched as one might think. We humans often make decisions that affect our entire life based on what can only be called anecdotes. Something happens once, and we make it guide our future decisions forever, especially if the event is vivid, recent, memorable, or all three. A swarthy curly-haired man in a BMW cuts me off rather dangerously at a road junction. I get scared and angry. I subconsciously conclude that swarthy curly-haired men in BMWs

---

*   I often have wondered what this represents in a court of law: beyond reasonable doubt or on the balance of probabilities? I think that it is somewhere between the two, but probably closer to the former. If any lawyer is reading this, please feel free to set me straight.

are all dangerous drivers. This is called the 'availability heuristic', or the example rule. Our minds are tuned to look for an example in memory and follow its findings and conclusions, rather than to ask the question: 'If this situation occurs 1,000 times, how likely is it that the outcome will be such and such?'*

Let us now go back to surgeons. If you hear that surgeon A has a mortality of 20 per cent and surgeon B has a mortality of 40 per cent, the first question you must ask is: how many patients are we talking about here? If it is only a handful of patients, the difference is due to chance. If it is a thousand patients each, we have a real difference (and, by the way, two surgeons to avoid absolutely, if the operation we are talking about is CABG).

Even after we have confirmed that the difference is statistically significant, we still need some more information before coming to any conclusion about how good or bad A and B are. Imagine that we have looked at the data for the two surgeons with different CABG mortality, and that we have ensured that the proper statistical tests have been applied. We have confirmed that their figures were derived from over a thousand patients each (large enough sample) and that the difference between the mortalities is also large enough to matter. The statistics tell us that the p-value on this difference is less than 0.05. In plain language, statistics say that the likelihood of finding a difference of *that* magnitude in *that* number of patients due to *chance alone* is less than 5 per cent. The conclusion that can be drawn about our two surgeons is inescapable: they do indeed have a difference in CABG mortality, and, this time, the difference is real. Can we conclude that the surgeon with the lower mortality is a better surgeon?

---

* That the example rule often deceives and misguides is explored beautifully in Dan Gardner's *Risk*. It is also ruthlessly exploited by peddlers of snake oil and alternative-medicine remedies.

The answer is still 'No'. The main reason for this is that our two surgeons could well be operating on very different patients. One surgeon may only take on young and relatively healthy patients with absolutely nothing wrong with them other than the heart problem. The other surgeon may be operating on very old patients with a weak heart muscle, diabetes, kidney failure, previous strokes, and damaged lungs. Other things being equal, you would certainly expect the latter group to have a higher mortality than the former, no matter who was doing the operation. The problem is that we did not, until fairly recently, have any objective way of assessing how old and sick the patients were. In other words, there was no easy way of telling the predicted risk of an operation in advance by looking at the features of the patient.

Naturally, there were always subjective ways of predicting the risk. Experienced doctors and surgeons have an eye for these things, so we could ask the surgeons themselves, but, in my experience, that is a terrible method of obtaining risk information. Ask any surgeon the question, 'Who in your hospital does the most difficult, challenging, and high-risk operations?' and the answer is very likely to be, 'Why, that would be me, of course!'

There are good (and not so good) reasons for surgeons to harbour these self-delusions. To some extent, surgeons in general and heart surgeons in particular need a lot of self-confidence to function. A heart surgeon, day after day, walks into an operating theatre, nonchalantly cracks open the chest, puts the patient on an artificial heart–lung machine, stops the heart, opens it, fixes it, starts it again, disconnects the patient from the heart–lung machine, and expects that the heart will handle supporting life again after this abuse. Self-doubt has never been a prominent feature in the heart surgeon's psychological make-up. In fact, it has been said that, if you ask any heart surgeon to name the three greatest heart surgeons who ever existed, he would struggle to find the names of the other two. Surgeons' opinions of their own prowess and of the risk profile of their patients are therefore not reliable, and certainly not objective. Can an objective method be found?

It can, and it was.

The year was 1989, and I had just been employed as a senior trainee in heart surgery in Sheffield, the city in the north of England once famed for steel manufacture, the decline of which was vividly illustrated in the hit film *The Full Monty*. In the Northern General Hospital, among the disused steel mills of Sheffield, I worked for a senior surgeon called Professor Geoffrey Smith, a normally placid, affable man, and, by all accounts, an easy boss to work for. Early one Monday morning, I had finished the rounds of the cardiac intensive care unit, and was in the staff common room enjoying a coffee and indulging my longstanding addiction to *The Guardian*'s cryptic crossword before the day's operating began. Geoffrey Smith burst into the room in an uncharacteristic state of obvious excitement, clutching some photocopied pieces of paper, which he handed to me, saying, 'I believe this is one of most important papers I have ever seen! Will you read it and tell me what you think?'

I tried, probably unsuccessfully, to conceal my deeply felt preference for the crossword and a bit of peace and quiet before going to the operating theatre, and picked up the research article. It was something he had dug out of a recently published supplement to the medical journal *Circulation*. The article was by Victor Parsonnet, a New Jersey cardiac surgeon, and his two collaborators, Bernstein and Dean, from the Newark Beth Israel Medical Center (Parsonnet 1989). It had the unwieldy title 'A Method of Uniform Stratification of Risk for Evaluating the Results of Surgery in Acquired Adult Heart Disease'. What Parsonnet did was so simple that it is remarkable that it had not been done earlier in medicine.

He gathered data on a few thousand patients having heart operations at his hospital. He found out what features in these patients, their heart condition, and their heart operations were linked to mortality from the operation. He assigned each factor a 'weight' depending on how likely it was that this factor would be associated with an outcome of death, and built a scoring system. The scoring system was 'additive': you took the risk factors that were present, and added their weights to come up with a number. This number, expressed as a percentage, tells you the likelihood of death after such an operation in such a patient. We call this the predicted mortality. For example, if the patient was female (1 point) and diabetic (3 points), the risk of CABG, according to the Parsonnet model, was 1 + 3 = 4 per cent.

Geoffrey Smith was right. This was a very important paper. The obvious immediate benefit of such a system was that it could help both the patient and the doctor come to a sensible decision about whether or not to go ahead with an operation. Less obviously, but perhaps more importantly, by providing an objective way of predicting the outcome, Parsonnet gave us a benchmark against which to compare the actual outcome. The paper had the potential of turning the world of heart surgery (and of medical practice in general) on its head. Doctors and nurses would, of course, continue to do their best for their patients, but now, for the first time ever, at least in this one specialty of heart surgery, we had a way of knowing how good that 'best' really was.

The risk factors that contribute to the Parsonnet score, and their 'weights', are listed opposite:

Risk Factor	Parsonnet Score[a]
female	1
obesity	3
diabetes	3
hypertension (> 140 mmHg)	3
ejection fraction (a measure of how well the left ventricle — the main heart pump — works)	
• > 50 per cent (good)	0
• 30–49 per cent (moderate)	2
• < 30 per cent (poor)	4
age	
• 70–74 years	7
• 75–79 years	12
• > 79 years	20
valve operation	5
valve + CABG	7
pulmonary hypertension (high blood pressure in the lungs)	3
intra-aortic balloon pump (having a device for supporting a weak heart)	2
previous heart operation	
• one	5
• two	10
on dialysis for kidney failure	10
catheter lab emergency	10
catastrophic states	10–50 to be decided by the surgical resident
a few other rare factors	to be decided by the surgical resident

Parsonnet and colleagues went on to give an interpretation, with a somewhat arbitrary grouping of patients into risk categories from 'good' risk to 'extremely high' risk, as in the table below:

Parsonnet Score	Risk
0–4	good
5–9	fair
10–14	poor
15–19	high
20+	extremely high

Knowing what we now know about risk modelling, there are a few features of the Parsonnet model that can be readily criticised. First, it was built from data obtained from a single hospital, so its widespread application may not be reliable. In fact, the model may well contain a biased reflection of the peculiarities of practice in that one institution. Second, as folk tried the model in their own units, many found that their own mortality rates were a lot smaller than Parsonnet predicted, so that the 'calibration' of the model may have been a little off-kilter: it overpredicted mortality. Perhaps, at the time, the results of heart surgery were not as good in Parsonnet's own unit as they should have been, or perhaps the model deliberately overstated the risks in order not to upset the medical establishment. Last, there were features in the model that left too much to subjective interpretation: for example, the definition of 'catastrophic state' or 'rare risk factors' could be awarded whatever risk value the surgical resident chose. This was neither rigorous nor objective, and it opened the model to the possibility of gaming.

Be that as it may, it would be churlish to criticise what was, in effect, a major groundbreaker. Parsonnet had created a model that made sense to his surgical colleagues, was intuitive, could reasonably predict outcomes, and could be applied by all. It was easy to use, and it was the first of its kind. The vital importance of this first step cannot be overstated: it opened the door to quality control in cardiac surgery, and that, in turn, ushered in quality control in medicine as a whole.

Surgeons are not, as a general rule, well known for their rapacious appetite for reading. An old medical joke goes like this:

Q: How do you hide money from an orthopaedic surgeon?
A: Put it in a medical textbook.
Q: How do you hide money from a general surgeon?
A: Put it in the patient's case notes.
Q: How do you hide money from a plastic surgeon?
A: You can't hide money from a plastic surgeon!

When surgeons actually do read scientific papers, it is often to find out how other surgeons do operations, to learn about newfangled operations, and to look at gory pictures.

The initial response to the publication of Parsonnet's paper lay somewhere between 'muted' and 'non-existent'. When it was first published, relatively few people read it, and even fewer, like Geoffrey Smith, appreciated its tremendous importance. To begin with, it had appeared in a specialist medical journal rather than in a dedicated surgical one. It also was fairly well hidden in a supplement, rather than appearing in the main journal itself. Finally, your average heart surgeon (who rarely reads *Circulation* anyway, and almost never reads the supplement) is unlikely to be fired with enthusiasm by a paper describing risk modelling (and with no gory pictures).

Slowly, however, the value of having a tool for predicting outcomes began to achieve the recognition it deserved. Some American hospitals tried the Parsonnet model in their own heart surgery practice, and found that it worked pretty well, and they published this finding in journals. Having shortly afterwards left Sheffield to work as a senior registrar in Manchester, I thought I would do the same in a British hospital. I collected the data on the Parsonnet risk factors in our patients, and used the information to see how well Parsonnet worked in a British hospital. At the time, the senior surgeons for whom I worked looked at my obsession with the subject with some degree of detached bemusement. I went on to publish the findings in the *British Medical Journal* (Nashef 1992) as the first application of the Parsonnet model in a British hospital, my own Wythenshawe Hospital in Manchester. Essentially, the study proved that a risk model from across the Atlantic worked pretty well in a British hospital, and that our results were actually better than the model predicted, so everybody was happy. Soon, other reports on clinical research in heart surgery would routinely begin by describing groups of patients in terms of average age, sex distribution, and Parsonnet score. The importance of measuring the risk profile of patients when reporting clinical results was at last being appreciated.

Much more importantly, Parsonnet gave us a way of predicting mortality, and, by doing so, he provided a benchmark: at last, we had something against which actual mortality could be assessed. In other words, surgeons who operated on widely varying patient groups in terms of risk could pitch their results against this benchmark.

4

Accurate Predictions

The original Parsonnet paper had achieved a respectable amount of impact, and my paper on the trial of the model in a British hospital had been well received. I was coming to the end of my specialty training, but there was still some more work to do before I would be ready to seek appointment as an independent surgeon, and that had to be something truly special, as the competition for the coveted posts of senior or consultant heart surgeon was (and still is) fierce. It was the last year of my training, and I had to choose an exceptional location in which truly special skills could be obtained. In those days, many senior medical trainees in the United Kingdom added the final lustre to the polish on their credentials by going to the United States to do research or some other attachment in their chosen specialty. In fact, so common was this practice that it acquired the unofficial status of a kind of additional qualification:

Mr Joe Hacker-Forceps

MB BS FRCS BTA

(Medical Bachelor, Bachelor of Surgery, Fellow of the Royal
College of Surgeons, Been To America)

I did not fancy seeking a BTA, largely because working in a laboratory and being told what research I could or could not do left me cold. I wanted an attachment with a bit more freedom, and with a focus on clinical work. The university hospitals of Bordeaux in France offered specialist areas in cardio-thoracic surgery and transplantation that were unique — on top of which, I already had some French connections, could speak the language, and was partial to a nice Margaux wine. So Bordeaux it was. It lived up to expectations. The pay was terrible, the work was hard, and the impact on my young family severe, but, in terms of the value of the clinical attachment, the place was unbeatable. Some of the best surgery I had ever seen took place there, and I made the most of the experience, not just by learning from the precise and meticulous way French surgeons did everything both in and out of the operating theatre, but also from the rich pickings that their advanced surgery offered for scientific publication. Many French doctors had a poor command of the English language and found it difficult to publish in the predominantly English-speaking medical world, and so I was able to offer my services as a medical writer and translator to get their work the recognition it so richly deserved in the mainstream Anglophone medical literature, while, at the same time, becoming a co-author on some innovative and high-profile clinical papers.

I therefore operated, learned, and wrote in Bordeaux, but I also befriended François Roques, an ambitious, intelligent, but somewhat surly senior trainee heart surgeon who was desperately looking to improve his own curriculum vitae by publishing something. 'So publish something', I said. 'Yes, it is easy for you to say, but what? It's all been done before', said François, and so I suggested risk modelling applied to French cardiac surgery, along the same lines of my then recent paper from Manchester on the Parsonnet score. At first, I was met with a blank stare. The concept of quality monitoring and risk assessment was not, at that time, common currency in France. After a few brief words of explanation, François's eyes lit up. He saw the value of such work, and decided to do it.

In fact, François Roques did a lot more than simply apply Parsonnet in France. He and his collaborators also modified the Parsonnet model to fit the French patient population, thus effectively creating their own French risk model, compared the two, and found that theirs was better. The paper describing this 'French score' was published in 1997. It had relatively little impact, because its appeal to the profession outside France was necessarily limited. By then, I was back in Britain, having achieved my career ambition and secured a consultant post. I was working at Papworth Hospital in Cambridge, one of the world's greatest institutions for cardiac surgery, when François unexpectedly got in touch. He, too, had become a consultant (*praticien hospitalier*), and was now working in Martinique in the French West Indies, but the balmy Caribbean environment had done nothing to dampen his newfound enthusiasm for risk modelling.

'I think you and I can do better', he said.

'Better than what?'

'Better than Parsonnet, better than the French score, better than everything. We should create our own risk model.'

I liked the sound of that, and the two of us agreed to go ahead.

Email was still not widely available at the time, so, over the next couple of years, the fax lines between Cambridge and Martinique were, we like to think, glowing red hot on the ocean bed with the enormous amount of data travelling through them, back and forth, as we argued over which risk factors to study, and over the shape and strategy of the project. We decided to collect data

from all over Europe. I belonged to the European Club of Young
Cardiac Surgeons, which met annually in a different European city,
and I was able to recruit my fellow club members to co-ordinate
the exercise in their own country. François and I picked out
every risk factor known or suspected to influence outcome. We
designed a user-friendly, single-sided A4 form to collect the data,
with carefully designed wording and explanations. We asked for
data on risk factors, the operation performed, and the outcome:
was the patient alive or dead afterwards? We even designed a logo
(dismissively described by my then secretary as looking like a
cheap shoe for a deformed foot):

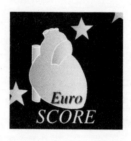

We printed out tens of thousands of these forms, packaged them,
and sent them to individual hospitals in eight European countries,
and recruited one of the best biostatisticians in France, Philippe
Michel, of the University of Bordeaux, to do the analysis. After all
the data were gathered, some 20,000 patients from 128 hospitals in
eight European countries were studied, and information collected
on 97 risk factors in all the patients. The data were laboriously
transcribed into a computer database at the University of Bordeaux.
We therefore knew the risk profile of the patients, and we knew
which had survived. We then flew to Bordeaux to create the risk
model. For days, Francois, Philippe, and I studied and validated data,
and designed and discarded models, and the university computers

churned the data and tested and tweaked each successive version of the possible models. Finally, at about two in the morning on 2 May 1997, we had a model that worked very well and was simple to use, intuitive, and credible. We named it the European System for Cardiac Operative Risk Evaluation (EuroSCORE), and, feeling chuffed with the elegant acronym, went to bed.*

The paper describing EuroSCORE was accepted for presentation at the plenary session of the next meeting of the European Association for Cardio-Thoracic Surgery in Brussels, and I had the privilege of reading the paper to a packed house. A few weeks later, the full paper was published in the association's journal (Nashef 1999).

The success of EuroSCORE exceeded our wildest expectations. The model has been used globally, in every continent and in almost every country with cardiac surgery. The paper alone has been cited in more than 2,300 scientific publications, and the term EuroSCORE has entered the medical vocabulary. The risk model that it refers to has been used for decision-making about the risk of surgery, for evaluating the quality of care, for predicting death (which it was designed to do), for comparing the results of surgery, for predicting complications (which it was not designed to do), and for estimating the cost and length of hospitalisation. In some countries, it has even entered the legal system, so that the family of a heart surgery patient with a low EuroSCORE is automatically compensated if he or she dies.

Now that we have a risk model, how do we put it into practice? When a risk model allows us to predict the likely outcome, we

---

* That's not strictly true. François and Philippe went to bed, and I went to my hotel room and switched on the BBC news to watch the gradual unfolding of the landslide that brought Tony Blair to power after nearly two decades of Conservative Party rule.

immediately have a benchmark against which we can compare the *actual* outcome. The easiest and most basic use of this tool is for the monitoring of surgical performance using hospital mortality (death from the operation).

Most patients admitted to hospital for a heart operation, or any other kind of operation, are alive when they enter hospital. Very rarely, a patient arrives 'dead but warm', and is brought back to life by a heart operation, but this is extremely rare. We can therefore safely assume that virtually all patients having a heart operation are alive when they come in to hospital, and most will be alive when they leave hospital after operation. The difference between the number coming in alive and the number leaving alive is the hospital mortality. This is an objective measure, difficult to falsify, and available in the data of almost any hospital, no matter how rudimentary the hospital information system. Thus the hospital mortality can be expressed as a percentage: if 100 patients enter the hospital alive, and 98 leave the hospital alive, then the *actual* mortality is 2 per cent.

A risk model such as EuroSCORE allows us to predict what that mortality should be on average, taking into account the risk profile of the patients. By adding up the EuroSCOREs for all 100 patients together, and dividing by 100, we have another percentage, and that is the average *predicted* mortality.

The next step is to compare the two. If a particular hospital's actual mortality is 1 per cent and its predicted mortality is 2 per cent, can we conclude that this hospital is doing better than predicted? No, we can't. We can be pretty sure that the hospital is doing *no worse* than predicted, but, to be able to say that it is actually doing *better* than predicted, we need to be confident that the result isn't likely to be due to chance.

When we look at data, we very rarely look at the entire data from the population that interests us. Most of the time, we collect a sample of data, and hope that the findings in that sample reflect those in the whole population. The reason is simple: it is usually difficult and time-consuming to measure anything in a whole population. Say, for example, you wanted to find out the average height of people in your town. You could line them all up and measure them, but that would take a huge effort and a very long time, especially if your town is London or Melbourne. Much easier would be to take a random sample of a few hundred folk in your town and measure them, and hope that your sample is representative of the whole population. How confident can you be that the measurement you took actually reflects the real average height of all the townsfolk? The statisticians have a very good method to answer that question, and that is what is called the 'confidence interval'. In a way, this is also analogous to decisions made in law. Like a judge asking a jury to be sure beyond reasonable doubt that the accused is guilty, stating the confidence interval gives us the range within which we can be certain beyond reasonable doubt that the true value of what we are interested in lies within that range. We now know that the arbitrary cut-off point for certainty in medicine is established. In medical statistics, to be beyond reasonable doubt is to be at least 95 per cent certain.

There is more than one method of working out the confidence interval, and the choice depends on the type of data one is dealing with. If you are measuring the height of people in a population, the distribution of these heights will be 'normal', or, in other words, it follows the well-known shape of the bell curve, with most measurements clustered around the average, and the rest becoming less and less frequent on either side of the average.

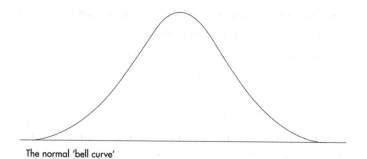

The normal 'bell curve'

Certain events, such as death after heart surgery, happen rarely, say 2 per cent of the time. If we look at many patient groups, and plot all the mortalities on a graph, we do not get a normal distribution, or a bell curve. Instead, we get a skewed distribution, with most measured mortalities clustered around 0–4 per cent, then a long and diminishing 'tail' of higher mortalities. This sort of distribution is called a Poisson distribution, named after the 19th-century French mathematician Siméon Poisson.

A crude representation of a Poisson distribution of mortalities is shown below:

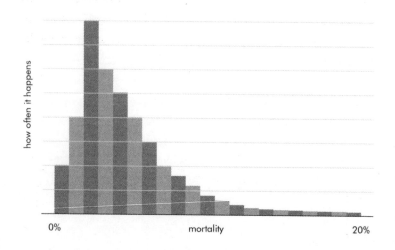

The important thing about the Poisson distribution is the longish tail, and that also applies to the confidence interval around a measurement that follows such a distribution.

So we have a measurement of mortality of 2 per cent in a decent sample of heart surgery patients. If we know the sample size, we can calculate that the 95 per cent confidence interval around this measurement is going to be, say, 1–4 per cent. This means that, based on our sample mortality of 2 per cent, we can be 95 per cent confident that the true mortality in the population will be between 1 and 4 per cent. The reason we need to know the sample size is simple. If the sample is large, we can be more confident that it will truly represent the population, and we will get a tighter confidence interval: say 1.5 to 3 per cent. If the sample is tiny (like the snake-oil salesman sample), we will have a hugely wide confidence interval, say 0.5 to 70 per cent, and our measure of 2 per cent would be meaningless.

Armed with this information, we can now use the measured sample mortality and the 95 per cent confidence interval properly and sensibly to compare outcomes. For that, take a look at these hypothetical scenarios. First, we take a surgeon whose mortality is 3 per cent, as shown by the diamond shape. EuroSCORE tells us his predicted mortality is 4 per cent, and that is shown by the vertical bar.

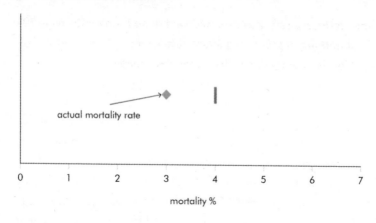

So, is this surgeon doing better than predicted? Maybe, but we will not know for sure until we apply the 95 per cent confidence interval, so let us do that:

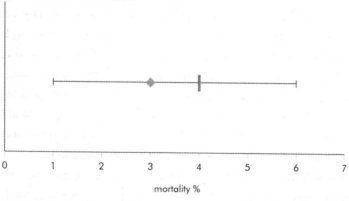

The horizontal bar around the diamond of actual mortality shows the 95 per cent confidence interval. It goes from 1 per cent to 6 per cent, which includes within its limits the predicted mortality of 4 per cent. Therefore we can be 95 per cent confident that based on our sample, the surgeon's true mortality is 1–6 per cent, no better and no worse than predicted. This surgeon is therefore performing as expected, and there is no reason to worry (and nothing to get excited about either!).

Now look at these four hypothetical surgeons:

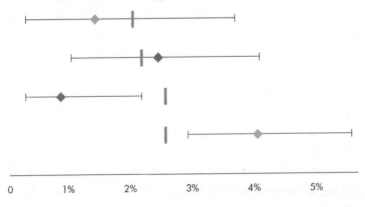

The top two are doing as well as predicted, in that there is no significant difference between their actual mortality (diamond) and their predicted mortality (vertical bar). We can say this because the predicted mortality lies within the 95 per cent confidence interval of their actual mortality (horizontal bar). The third is doing significantly better than predicted, and should perhaps be given a pay rise. The fourth is doing significantly worse, and needs some action now, before more patients suffer.

The above method is the statistically correct one for knowing if one surgeon (or unit, or service, or hospital) is performing as expected, better than expected, or less well than expected. There are other indicators, perhaps less statistically rigorous, but no less useful for that. To understand them, we shall pretend to be bankers (of the old-fashioned type that count your money and look after it, not the type that gamble with billions and cause global economic meltdown).

'The surgeon saved my mother's life!'

'The surgeon killed my mother!'

Both of the above are sensationalist statements, and, in the overwhelming majority of cases, both are utterly wrong. Surgeons almost never save a whole life, and almost never kill an entire mother. They do, however, save and lose 'bits' of a life. Let me explain.

No operation has zero risk. In fact, no medical procedure or treatment has zero risk. A single aspirin tablet is capable of provoking a stomach bleed or an allergic reaction that can be fatal. In fact, eating just one peanut can be fatal if you have a peanut allergy, and a peanut is not even a medicine. Crossing the road, getting out of bed, and getting into bed with the wrong partner can all kill you. An average female patient having a CABG operation in the current era has a risk of dying of approximately 1 per cent. If she dies, can her son blame the surgeon? Well, yes, but not entirely. He can blame the surgeon for 99 per cent of her death, but that 1 per cent was always on the cards, no matter who the surgeon was or what the surgeon did.

Similarly, if the woman survives, can the surgeon take the credit for saving her life? Well, yes, but not entirely. In fact, there was a 99 per cent chance she would survive anyway, no matter who the surgeon was. The surgeon can, however, justifiably take the (minuscule) credit for that paltry 1 per cent of a life saved, and this brings us to the 'bank of life'.

Imagine a bank in which we deposit not money, but lives, or parts of lives. Every surgeon has a bank account. When a patient survives an operation, the account gets a credit equal to the probability of death from the operation. Similarly, when a patient dies from an operation, the account is debited by the probability of survival.

Let us now look at what this account balance sheet would look like in graphical form.

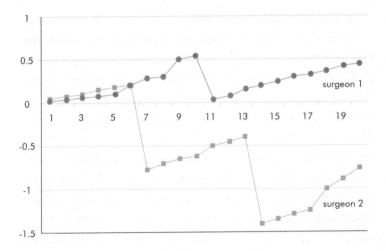

In this graph, we have two surgeons: surgeon 1 (line with circle dots) and surgeon 2 (line with square dots). On the horizontal axis, we have the total number of operations over time, and, in this graph, each surgeon has done 20 operations. On the vertical axis, we have the total number of lives 'saved' or, if you dip below the zero, lives 'lost'.

To begin with, until they reach patient number 6, both surgeons are doing pretty well. All their patients are surviving, but all of their patients have a low risk of death anyway, so the account is credited with tiny 'bits of life saved'. Note that when surgeon 1 operates on patient number 8, his line swings more sharply upwards. Patient number 8 was a high-risk patient (probability of death 25 per cent), so that surgeon 1 gets a whole 'quarter of a life' credited in one fell swoop. When he reaches patient number 10, another very high-risk patient, unfortunately the patient dies, but as the probability of survival for this patient was only 50 per cent anyway, the account is only debited by half a life, and surgeon 1 continues on his upwards trend afterwards.

It is a completely different story for surgeon 2. He too is doing well until patient 6, but here the patient dies. Unfortunately, however, this was a low-risk patient, with a probability of survival of 95 per cent, so that almost a whole life (0.95 of one) is debited when that patient dies. This tragedy happens again at patient 13. The two line graphs now show clearly which surgeon is doing better.

This ingenious method was described by Jocelyn Lovegrove and colleagues from University College, London (Lovegrove 1997). The beauty of it is that an enormous quantity of data (numbers of operations, survival and death, risk profile, and how they all fare over a period of time) can be seen at a glance from a simple single-line diagram. One quick look at the diagram for a particular surgeon can give a pretty good estimate of performance by looking at risk-adjusted survival over time. In simple terms, the graph says to the surgeon: 'My friend, *this* is how well you've been doing' (or how badly). It is one of the most useful performance measures there has ever been, and all one needs to compile the graph are numbers of operations, patients' risk profile using EuroSCORE or some other method, and what the outcome was (dead or alive).

The method is called either the CuSum (cumulative sum) curve or sometimes VLAD (variable life-adjusted display, not Vlad the Impaler). Good institutions have data on the results achieved by their surgeons, and provide these data and graphs to them on a regular basis, and that, by taking advantage of an amazing phenomenon called the Hawthorne effect, is probably the single most important measure by which the results of medical intervention can be sustained and improved.

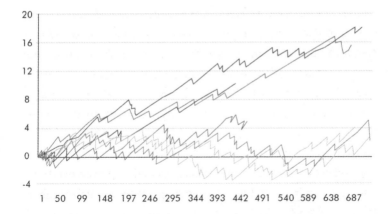

A real VLAD or CuSum curve for Papworth Hospital in Cambridge. Three surgeons are doing superbly well. Four are doing as expected, though, for a short time, three dipped below the zero in the 'lives saved' account. They were only overdrawn for a very short time, and rapidly got back to safety. Interestingly, one of them was going through an acrimonious divorce at the time, and was not concentrating on his work, and his results suffered. Another was going through an overconfident phase, was very pleased with himself, and thought he could get away with anything. He took some risks, and his results suffered. As we will see later, the psychology of surgeons (who are, after all, human beings, despite claims to the contrary) can have an impact on outcomes.

The success of EuroSCORE in becoming the world's leading risk model went far beyond its use in medical decision-making and quality control. It actually saved lives. To understand how a mere risk model can do this, we have to go back to the early 20th century, and specifically to Cicero in Illinois, USA, home of the Hawthorne Works.

The Hawthorne Works was a factory complex built by the Western Electric Company in 1905. It had 45,000 employees at the height of its operations, making refrigerators and other electrical goods. In its heyday, it was so large that it had its own private railway to move shipments through the plant to the nearby freight depot. Sadly, in 1983, manufacturing ceased, and the plant became yet another shopping centre, but not before having secured a prominent place in history. That accolade, by the way, had absolutely nothing to do with making vacuum cleaners and refrigerators.

In the 1920s, some highly clever managers at the Hawthorne Works decided to study efficiency at the factory. They wondered whether the workers would be more productive if the ambient lighting in the factory was increased, so they turned up the lighting and measured the workers' productivity. They found that productivity temporarily increased, and, being managers, they were very pleased with themselves.

Some time later, the very same managers postulated that productivity should go down if lighting was reduced, so they turned down the lights and measured productivity. To their surprise, productivity went up. They were baffled by this unexpected finding. They pressed on, and studied the effect of many other interventions on productivity: raising and lowering the ambient temperature, moving desks around, meaninglessly changing the order in which routine tasks were carried out, and so on. Every time they implemented a change, they measured productivity and found that it went up for a while, only to return to baseline when the experiment stopped. Eventually, in 1932, they stopped intervening (much to the relief of the workers, I imagine), and filed their results.

Twenty years later, in the 1950s, a social scientist named Henry A. Landsberger revisited the Hawthorne experiments. Having studied the data, Landsberger had a brilliant idea. He postulated that the increased productivity may have had nothing to do with lights, temperature, or position of desks, but that it was the act of measurement itself that was improving the performance (Landsberger 1958). This phenomenon became known as the Hawthorne effect: in other words, measure something, and it gets better. Though puzzling at first, it is easy, on a little reflection, to see why mere measurement is capable of improving performance.

First, workers are human. If they perceive that somebody somewhere is interested in their performance, they are naturally motivated to improve. Second, where there is no measurement, there is absolutely no incentive to improve: if a factory, or a hospital for that matter, is underperforming, but is not measuring its performance, and not comparing itself to similar organisations or institutions, it cannot be aware of the existence of an underperformance problem, and the impetus for fixing the problem simply does not exist. If the old adage says 'If it ain't broke, don't fix it', then a corollary would go 'If you don't even know it's broke, why on Earth would you wanna try to fix it?' This was, almost certainly, at least part of the problem in children's heart surgery at the Bristol Royal Infirmary, as it probably was and unfortunately still is in many medical services around the world.

With the introduction of EuroSCORE to predict the mortality of surgery with reasonable accuracy, surgeons at last had a standard against which they could assess their own performance. They were no longer in the dark when it came to knowing how well or badly they were doing. The Hawthorne effect swung into action, and the inevitable happened. The results of cardiac surgery improved worldwide, and the greatest improvements were seen in those countries that had the most robust measurement systems. As a cause-and-effect phenomenon, this is impossible to prove. As a general rule, medicine, like everything else, gets better

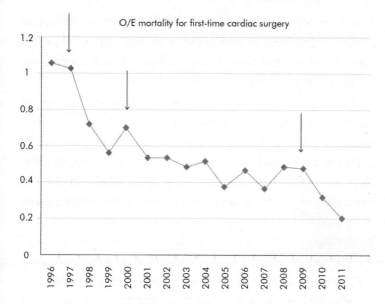

The ratio between observed (O) and expected (E) mortality at Papworth over the period during which risk models were introduced. The lower the line, the lower is the mortality (taking account of the risk profile). Each of the three arrows marks the introduction of a risk model: in 1997, Parsonnet; in 2000, EuroSCORE; and, in 2009, a tighter, modified EuroSCORE. Every single initiative was followed by a sharp drop in mortality.

Of course, for us makers of risk models, one of the downsides of the Hawthorne effect is that the risk model responsible for the improvement in outcomes falls victim to its own success. As a direct result of the better survival that follows its application for monitoring, the model becomes wildly inaccurate. By 2005, reports were trickling from some institutions that actual mortality was a lot lower than the EuroSCORE model predicted. During the following two to three years, the trickle became a flood. The model was still excellent at distinguishing between a low-risk and a high-risk patient, but its ability to measure the magnitude of that risk was inaccurate across the board. There was nothing to do but create another model, and that is exactly what we did. François Roques and I formed a new team to work on this venture, and were joined by Linda Sharples, then Medical Research Council statistician in Cambridge, now Professor of Statistics in Leeds. We collected data on more than 20,000 patients from hundreds of hospitals in over 50 countries of all continents, and recreated the model with contemporary data (Nashef 2012). This model (EuroSCORE II) is now available, and early signs indicate that the cardiac surgical community has adopted it enthusiastically.

One of the tasks of the EuroSCORE II project was to find out what exactly is a death. This is not a facetious comment: I alluded earlier to the fact that, after an operation, even death can be difficult to define. The following can all, with varying degrees of legitimacy, lay claim to the title 'early postoperative death'. If the patient dies on the operating table, there is no argument: it is an operative death. If the patient survives the operation, but dies two days later, most people would agree that this is an 'early' or postoperative death. We can also define survival or death as the state that the patient is in when leaving the hospital after an operation, as this is clear and cannot be argued with, but what if the patient never leaves hospital, and goes on to die in hospital six years after an operation? Is that still a postoperative or early death? An alternative would be to say the patient is considered to have survived the operation if he or she is still alive 30 days after the operation, but even that has problems.

First, it is not much use to the patient if an operation results in complications, and the patient stays on the intensive care unit being supported by increasingly desperate measures and expensive high-tech equipment, until death occurs on day 31. Second, some patients go home and die a few days later, but by then they are no longer under the beady eye of the hospital audit department, and whoever is collecting the mortality data may never find out about the tragic events that can happen after hospital discharge. This is further complicated by the fact that many people, like Professor Paul Sergeant of Leuven in Belgium, believe, with good justification from survival data, that the true attrition rate for death after an operation does not truly level out until 90 days after an operation, not 30 days. Ninety days is an awfully long time for an audit department to track the patients, some of whom may have moved house, emigrated, or simply no longer want to stay in touch with their treating hospital because they have better things to do. Hospitals, like all organisations, are not awash with money, and many other priorities compete for their limited resources with greater clamour than the chasing of old patients around the country and beyond to see how they have fared after leaving hospital.

We therefore looked at the data that the hospitals gave us in the EuroSCORE II study, and found that all hospitals could give us 100 per cent of the data on the status of the patient on leaving hospital (dead or alive). When it came to 30 days, just over half the hospitals had data. When it came to 90 days, the proportion dropped to below half. We therefore took a drastic decision, and defined an early death as one that occurs in the same hospital during the same admission as the operation. This was arbitrary and pragmatic: these data we knew were both available and accurate, important features to consider when one chooses a benchmark. We can still learn valuable lessons from those hospitals that actually had data on patients after they left hospital. These data were very valuable in that they helped us to find out what was the attrition rate after discharge from hospital: we found that, if the mortality is 4 per cent, at 30 days it rises by another 0.6 per cent and, at 90 days, by another 0.9 per cent. As we know that the rate levels off afterwards, we can postulate that these additional risks should be proportionately taken into account when you decide to have an operation. A little risk still lingers up to 90 days, and thereafter you are probably safe. This is something to bear in mind if you ever find yourself contemplating an operation and weighing up the risks versus the benefit: most of the risk will be concentrated in the time you are an in-patient in hospital, but there is still a little bit left to go through after you go home, and this levels out when you reach 90 days.

Heart surgery today mostly has its house in order. There are at last robust and objective monitoring tools to measure the quality of surgery, even if they simply focus on the relatively crude outcome of survival. These tools are sufficient to detect underperformance, and can provide the information and impetus necessary to correct such underperformance. In the current era, a poor hospital or a rogue surgeon with terrible results will be either corrected or stopped from operating. In the United Kingdom and in many other countries, data on outcomes are routinely measured, and action is taken as soon as the data indicate substandard performance. If you seek the treatment of heart surgery for yourself or a loved one in the United Kingdom, you may not receive the best in the country, but you will certainly receive treatment that is up to a high international standard regardless of which hospital or surgeon you choose, and that is surely a comforting thought. Similar monitoring in other countries also goes a long way to ensure that heart surgery there is also likely to be of a safe standard.* In general, the more robust is

---

* For instance, using AusSCORE and CuSum in Australia, or the STS score in North America.

the monitoring system, the safer is the surgery. Other surgical and medical specialties do not at present have anything like the level of monitoring that heart surgery has, but they are most certainly working, with varying degrees of reluctance, towards developing similar systems. My prediction is that it will not be long before all medical specialties will have robust monitoring and outcome measurements, and, when that happens, the Hawthorne effect will come into action, and the results and success of intervention in these specialties are likely to show a similar quantum leap in performance to that seen in heart surgery.

As well as saving tens of thousands of lives, a simple risk model such as EuroSCORE can have many direct uses. It can, for example, detect a doctor's underperformance, and may even stop a murderer in his tracks!

Like many other countries, Britain has seen its share of serial killers over the years. Around 1890, the so-called 'Jack the Ripper' gruesomely killed at least five women around the Whitechapel area in East London. Perhaps a few more murders were also indeed committed by him, but that has never been confirmed because of suspicion of copycat murders by other disturbed individuals who may have admired his handiwork. In the 1960s, Ian Brady and Myra Hindley, the infamous 'Moors Murderers', killed five children and buried them on Saddleworth Moor in Greater Manchester. The notorious Frederick West, later assisted by his wife Rosemary, went on a rape, torture, and killing spree that lasted nearly 20 years and resulted in the deaths of at least 11 young women. Horrific as all of these murderers were, their victim toll pales into insignificance when compared with Britain's most prolific serial killer of all time, a mild-mannered, and, by all accounts, respected and popular family doctor called Harold Shipman.

Dr Shipman was convicted for 15 proven murders over a

period spanning 25 years that only ended in 1998, but he is reliably believed to have murdered more than 250 people. This is many, many more than the Ripper, the Moors Murderers, and the Wests put together. For unfathomable reasons, Shipman killed hundreds of his own patients in their own homes or in his surgery, often by injecting them with lethal doses of diamorphine (the medical term for heroin). He signed their death certificates himself, giving spurious medical causes for their demise. Despite this huge death toll, he continued to practise medicine undetected for a quarter of a century. How could this have happened in a supposedly well-regulated profession such as medicine?

At the conclusion of the final report of the inquiry into the Shipman case, the High Court Judge Dame Janet Smith specifically pointed out that there was nothing unusual in Shipman's medical practice, such as the age and health (or otherwise) of his patients, that could possibly have explained why he had such a high death rate. Unfortunately, this observation came after the fact: until then, very little attention was paid to general practitioners in terms of measuring the mortality rates of their patients.

Following the inquiry report, an editorial comment was published in the medical journal *Anaesthesia*. In this editorial, the author (blessed with the somewhat unfortunate name of Dr Harmer) claimed that what happened with Shipman in general practice could not possibly happen in an NHS hospital. Dr Harmer argued that, in hospitals, doctors work in a highly regulated environment, with the slightest misdemeanour becoming common knowledge in a very short time, so that a serial killer like Dr Shipman could not possibly succeed in 'covering his tracks' in a modern hospital setting. My colleague Joe Arrowsmith, a consultant anaesthetist, read this editorial and was intrigued. Is it true that we would have detected a serial killer like Shipman if he was let loose in a hospital like Papworth?

Papworth Hospital already had fairly robust quality-measuring systems. One of the things we measured was risk-adjusted mortality for heart surgery. We compared our performance against EuroSCORE, and had a 'trip-wire': a metaphorical alarm bell would ring if any surgeon or anaesthetist had an actual mortality that was significantly greater than predicted by EuroSCORE.* This was the standard statistical test, and any surgeon or anaesthetist who 'rang the alarm bell' would be stopped and investigated. We also monitored all surgeons and anaesthetists using VLAD curves. These are not strictly statistical, but give a visual image of risk-adjusted performance over time. With these measures already in place, it was relatively easy to put the Shipman question to the test.

Joe Arrowsmith and I picked on two other colleagues as imaginary suspects (John Kneeshaw, an anaesthetist, and Stephen Large, a surgeon, who has also written an appendix to this book). Both had worked at Papworth for a long time, and had treated thousands of patients, with survival rates that were close to the average at Papworth. We turned them into virtual serial killers by developing a computer programme called Mock Unexpected Random Death Event Rate generator, an appropriate but gruesome acronym. The MURDER generator programme then randomly selected patients who were treated successfully by John and Steve, and 'reversed' the outcome. In other words, the computer pretended that these patients had died as a result of the treatment. We programmed it to 'kill' patients at random and at about the same rate that Shipman had done over his 25-year homicidal

---

* In this context, 'significantly' means that the statistics confirm that the probability of a mortality this much higher than EuroSCORE occurring due to chance and chance alone is less than 5 per cent, or, in other words, the p-value is less than 0.05.

career. We then applied our standard statistics to see how long it would have taken for either of them to ring the alarm bell and be stopped in their tracks.

The results of the experiment were outstanding (Arrowsmith 2006). Dr Harold Shipman went undetected for 25 years, and could have conceivably gone on killing had he not become careless. In our experiment, John, the anaesthetist, was picked up after ten months, and Steve, the surgeon, was picked up even quicker, within eight months. This was purely on the basis of their patients' death rates reaching statistical significance (in other words, a less than 5 per cent possibility of these occurring by chance). When we looked at the VLAD curves, both would have raised eyebrows and concern even earlier (see figure), probably in a matter of two to three months.

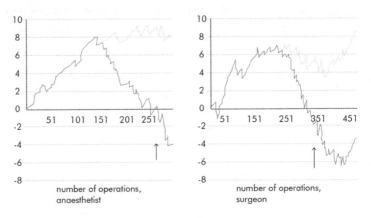

VLAD curves for serial-killer anaesthetist and surgeon. The killing starts when the curves branch out. The higher line is the true VLAD curve, the lower line is what happens to it had either of the two turned into Shipman. The arrow demonstrates when the statistical alarm bell is tripped (ten months for the anaesthetist and eight months for the surgeon), but the curves would have indicated a problem even earlier.

It is important to emphasise here that this was a fictitious scenario: both Steve and John are fine doctors with very good results. Ours was purely a computer simulation, designed to show what would happen *if* there was a serial killer at Papworth. There were no murders, and this simple fact was very clearly stated in the published article in *Anaesthesia*. Somehow, this obvious fact was not fully understood by all the tabloid newspapers, with one reporting that a serial killer went undetected at Papworth Hospital for eight months.

Of course, our quality-monitoring systems are not designed to detect serial killers, but are there to detect underperformance from any cause. What our study elegantly demonstrates is that such monitoring systems actually work. It makes a compelling argument for robust monitoring of outcomes in all hospitals, all operations, and all medical treatments in general. If we in the medical profession expect members of the public to trust us with their lives and the lives of their loved ones, then this is the least we should do.

5

Better Out of FIASCO

We often hear comparisons between surgeons and pilots (your life in their hands and all that). This has always struck me as somewhat superficial, because there are enormous differences between the two professions. For a start, a pilot flies an aeroplane, whereas a surgeon cuts people with a knife ('very, very carefully', according to my daughter Claudia, then aged five). An important similarity is that, of course, members of the public are usually prepared to place their trust — indeed lives — in the hands of pilots and surgeons alike. We rightly expect both pilots and surgeons to do their job 'very, very carefully', but there the similarities stop. On the one hand, the pilot is actually in the same boat (or aeroplane, to be literal) as the passengers. If the plane crashes and everybody dies, so does the pilot. A surgeon, on the other hand, will survive any number of his or her patients' 'crashes'. The surgeon's reputation and career may not survive, but the surgeon almost certainly will. A surgeon takes risks with the lives of others. A pilot risks his or her own life. An even more important distinction between a surgeon and a pilot is that they are radically different in their modus operandi.

A few years ago, I thought that I would try to train for a private pilot's licence. I had romantic delusions about flying to France for lunch, and the more prosaic notion that when I needed to travel somewhere quickly for a meeting, it would be easy and relatively inexpensive to charter a single-engine Cessna and go anywhere in the country without ever again having to endure the appalling degradation of flying with Ryanair. I also thought it would be cool. It was a short-lived venture. In the end, I gave it all up after half a dozen lessons, having learned to take off and to cruise but not yet to land. The reason for this was that aviation safety meant that I simply did not have enough time. The first flying lesson took an hour, and was fine. The second was preceded by a safety briefing that lasted 20 minutes. The third had a briefing and a debriefing. The fourth added safety checks to the briefing and debriefing. By the fifth lesson, I also had to become something of an amateur aircraft mechanic, checking obscure bits of the engine and fuel systems, and the supposed one-hour lesson was taking all day. From that ephemeral venture into aviation, however, I learned one of the biggest differences between pilots and surgeons. Pilots follow procedure, check and recheck, and then check again. They do their utmost to avoid leaving anything to chance. It's a belt-and-braces hold-on-to-your-pants-with-both-hands-just-in-case approach. Surgeons, in comparison with pilots, are gung-ho wide-eyed cowboys.

Two examples from heart surgery illustrate the point. Surgeons join most blood vessels using a single-filament suture made out of polypropylene. The suture is usually Prolene, a brandname product made by Ethicon, an international suture-manufacturing company. Prolene has many interesting features, some of which are good and some of which are bad. It is blue in colour, which is ridiculous, as it often becomes invisible against the ubiquitous blue background of the sterile operating-theatre drapes; and it has the handling characteristics of pubic hair, being both crinkly and unwieldy.

Despite these disadvantages, Prolene is the preferred suture worldwide for joining up blood vessels. There are three main reasons for this. First, it is slippery, so it glides through tissue swiftly and smoothly without causing damage. Second, it is inert, and the body happily accepts it; there is no evidence that it causes inflammation or any other adverse reaction in the tissues. Third (and most important), it is very strong, and retains its strength more or less forever. Blood vessels carefully sutured or joined with Prolene can withstand high arterial blood pressure, even when the calibre of the Prolene suture is so small as to be finer than a human hair. In a quadruple coronary bypass operation, there will be at least seven suture lines where a Prolene suture is the only structure protecting the patient from fatal bleeding. It is, literally, the thin blue line between life and death.

There are, however, two features of a Prolene suture that should modify the behaviour of surgeons when they are handling it. The first is that Prolene is slippery. The downside of its smooth passage through tissue is that a knot made out of it can slip if not properly 'locked'. To lock a knotted suture requires either a change of hands or a slight change in hand position while tying the knot, not exactly an arduous task. There are about three or four manoeuvres that will securely lock a knot, and all surgeons are aware of at least two of them. Careful surgeons begin by tying a number of slipknots, anything between four and seven. The slip allows the knot to be tightened to the desired firmness. They then do one of the available manoeuvres to lock the knot securely. In terms of time, the locking manoeuvre adds between half a second to three seconds to the procedure. In most operations on the heart and major blood vessels, a single running Prolene suture is used for joining and repairing blood-containing structures, including arteries that hold blood under high pressure, such as the aorta, which carries the entire blood output of the heart within its walls. So the slipping of a knot on the aorta can lead to the unravelling of an entire suture line and the patient bleeding to death in a matter of minutes. Knowing this, you would have thought that all surgeons would lock a Prolene knot, especially on an artery, and even more so if the artery happens to be the aorta. The shocking truth is that they do not. Of the surgeons I know, fewer than half properly lock every Prolene knot, even on an artery, even on the aorta itself.

The second drawback of Prolene is that it is a monofilament. Most strings in everyday use, such as the cotton you sew a garment with, the mooring line for a boat, or your shoelaces, are braided or multifilament: the string or rope is made up of several smaller strings entwined about each other. Some sutures other than Prolene are also braided or multifilament. The main advantage of a braided suture is that a fracture of one of its tiny strands does not jeopardise the integrity and strength of the whole suture. Prolene is different. It consists of merely one strand of material. In fact, if you look at Prolene under a powerful magnifying glass, all you will see is a single shiny, smooth, blue cylinder. A fracture of this one filament weakens or breaks the entire suture. So the manufacturers quite rightly advise against handling the suture with metal instruments such as surgical forceps, clips, or clamps for fear that a crack or fracture might weaken the suture, causing it to snap and (being slippery) unravel so that an entire suture line risks coming undone. Knowing this, you would have thought that no surgeons in their right minds would dream of touching a Prolene suture with metal forceps, or applying a metal clip or a clamp to it. The shocking truth is that most surgeons do, even if that suture is being used to repair an artery, and even if that artery is the aorta itself.

Fortunately, most multiple slipknots do not actually slip, and most Prolene somehow survives the assault of metal instruments, but not all. Over a 20-year career, I have personally seen a handful of patients bleed out and die from slipped knots and fractured Prolene. One was a man who was sipping his morning cup of tea after a successful CABG, when he bled out into the chest drains and died in a couple of minutes before anything could be done to retrieve the situation. Post-mortem examination showed that one of the joins of the coronary bypass had come undone because the Prolene was fractured. A metal clamp had been applied to it during the operation. Another was a man who had survived a difficult and high-risk heart transplant, only to collapse two hours later, having bled from an unravelled suture on the right atrium, a chamber of the heart. The team had got to him in time to re-open the chest, stop the bleeding, and massively transfuse him, but it was too late: he was brain dead. When his chest was re-opened, lying in a corner of the membrane enclosing the heart was an accusing, finger-pointing little blue twisted thread: the slipped Prolene suture, which had not been locked.*

The numbers of such calamities are minuscule, but even one is too many when the safety step required to avoid it is so simple and quick. Take a few extra seconds to lock a Prolene knot securely, and handle the Prolene with gloved fingers only or, if you must, with metal instruments whose sharpness is tempered by a rubber sheath (so-called rubber-shod forceps), and these calamities will never happen. The two surgeons involved in

---

* That unfortunate patient became an organ donor, and his kidneys and liver were taken for transplantation to others.

these cases learned their lesson the hard way, and now always lock sutures and never handle Prolene with metal. A third, a colourful and engaging bon vivant who was one of the greatest heart surgeons in Britain, was a supremely confident operator, thinker, and innovator. He had excellent clinical outcomes, and won the respect and admiration of the medical establishment in Britain and internationally. He was not shy of publicity, and at one point in his career came as close to being a 'household name' as any could in this profession. He, too, had a near miss, of a similar nature, when a slipped Prolene knot on the aorta unravelled a few hours after an operation. He managed by the skin of his teeth to save the patient from death by blood loss. He nevertheless continued his merry practice of not locking slipknots until his eventual retirement a few years ago.

In an era where we are supposed to be doing everything possible to make surgery safer, to reduce to the best of our ability the potential and actual harm to patients, and to strive endlessly to improve results, basic safety steps are not being taken. A large part of the reason is that surgeons are natural risk-takers. They occasionally cut corners, often make decisions on the hoof, and tend to act in a cavalier way. The obsessive and self-examining culture that prevails in aviation has not yet taken hold in the field of surgery. In aviation, all possible care is taken all the time. In medicine, as the following study demonstrates, it is not.

Recently, one of my colleagues, Catherine Sudarshan, decided to look into the care of Jehovah's Witnesses having major heart operations. Jehovah's Witnesses are a broadly Christian denomination, but with several beliefs that distinguish them from the mainstream, including the rejection of festivals such as Easter and Christmas as essentially pagan, and the belief that the Kingdom of God was established in October 1914 and has room for only 144,000 believers. From the point of view of a heart surgeon such as Catherine, the most important attribute of Jehovah's Witnesses is that they absolutely reject blood transfusion. For obvious reasons, blood transfusion can be essential for heart operations. In the early days of heart surgery, hardly an operation was carried out without the need for blood transfusion, and often in huge quantities. As we have got better at it, and our machines have become more sophisticated and compact, we have reached the stage where only around a third of patients need to be given any blood at all. A third, however, is a large minority, and the risk of needing at least some blood or blood products is very real.

A heart surgeon's own heart usually sinks when a Jehovah's Witness enters the consulting room. A patient who categorically refuses to have a blood transfusion takes one potential safety net away from the operation, and the surgeon knows that if major bleeding occurs during or after the operation, death is likely to follow. Some surgeons flatly refuse to operate on these patients, and most would refuse if they considered it likely that the proposed operation would result in excess bleeding. Catherine wanted to see what happens when Jehovah's Witnesses are operated on. Do they do worse than those patients who are prepared to accept blood? In other words, does the removal of the safety net actually damage them?

She studied all the Jehovah's Witnesses who received major heart operations at Papworth Hospital in the past few years, and found that they actually do not fare worse than other patients. There was no difference in their risk-adjusted mortality, and, overall, their cardiac outcomes were similar. In one important area, however, they actually did better than the others: they lost a lot less blood. The average blood loss in Jehovah's Witnesses was a mere 272 millilitres 12 hours after surgery. Other patients had an average blood loss of nearly double that (498 millilitres). What is happening here is obvious: because the patients refused blood transfusion, the surgeons must have taken more care to control bleeding. This begs the question: if it is possible to take more care with Jehovah's Witnesses, should we not take more care with everybody?

Common to both aviation and medicine is the concept of the near miss. It also demonstrates beautifully why surgeons are nothing like pilots. All it takes to constitute a near miss in aviation is for two planes to come reasonably close to each other so that an accident may have been possible. In aviation, therefore, a near miss is just that: an accident that could have happened but absolutely did not. In medicine, however, there are three types of near miss, which I classified in an article in *The Lancet* (Nashef 2003). In type 1, a mistake is made, the systems designed to detect it and correct it work as planned, and nothing happens. In type 2, the error is made and the safety systems fail, but no harm is done thanks to sheer luck alone. In type 3, harm is done, but it falls short of a direct hit — death or disability, or whatever is the outcome that is being studied. Near misses in aviation are overwhelmingly type 1, far more benign in nature than many near misses in medicine, and yet the aviation industry approaches them with absolute earnestness. All near misses are reported, collected, and scrupulously analysed. Lessons are learned from them, and changes in practice and protocol are introduced as a result. After all, it is so much safer (and more intelligent) to learn from a near miss than from a direct hit. Owing to near-miss observations and other technological improvements, the current rate of fatal accidents in air travel has dropped by about 65 per cent, to one fatal accident in about 4.5 million aeroplane departures, from one in nearly 2 million in 1997. We have no such systems in medicine. With occasional exceptions in the fields of drug prescription and blood transfusion, near-miss reporting is still in its infancy. There is some near-miss reporting in some surgical specialties, but in others it is almost non-existent, and in medical specialties it is totally non-existent. In clinical practice, on the whole, we are sadly still in the rudimentary stages of learning from a direct hit.

I never imagined that while working on this chapter about the medical profession's inability to learn from a near miss, a catastrophic event in my own practice would poignantly and viciously throw the issue into unforgivingly sharp focus.

One afternoon, I was operating on a 73-year-old woman with a narrowed aortic valve. The plan was to replace the valve with one made from animal tissue, with a view to relieving her breathlessness and reducing her chances of heart failure. The patient had a few risk factors, but nothing prohibitive, and we expected the operation to be smooth, quick, and relatively easy.

We attached the patient to the heart–lung machine in the usual way, and I inserted a tube into the left ventricle to keep the field free of blood while I replaced the valve. This tube was supposed to suck any blood from the ventricle, but, unfortunately on this occasion, it did not suck: it blew. The heart was filled with air, which went to the brain, and the patient suffered catastrophic and irreversible brain damage from which she died. Someone in the vicinity of the heart–lung machine must have unwittingly pushed the button that reversed the direction of the pump, so that instead of sucking blood away from the heart, it pumped air into the heart. Needless to say, this was an avoidable catastrophe, and a direct hit. The entire hospital immediately swung into action to study the root cause of the problem and see what could be learned from it. What we found was that it was ridiculously easy to reverse the pump accidentally: all it took was for an object, a finger, or an elbow to touch one sensitive button on the machine, and that made it blow instead of suck. On a human level, this was an unmitigated disaster for the patient and her loving family. On a professional level, it was a direct hit from which lessons could be learned, but I could not stop thinking how easily the accident had happened, and being somewhat surprised that it hadn't happened before.

In 20 years of working at the same hospital, I had not seen such a calamity until now, and this begged the question: if this event was the direct hit, was it preceded by any near misses? I asked the perfusionists and surgeons if they had ever witnessed such an accidental pump reversal before. To my horror, most said 'Yes'. All of them had seen it or, at the very least, were aware of it happening to colleagues, but, by sheer luck, on these past occasions the patients escaped injury: the archetypal type 2 near miss.

Within a few days, all staff at Papworth had been warned of the danger, and shown how the mistake could happen. Plans have already been implemented to change the operating procedures for this equipment pending either a modification of the design or the wholesale replacement of the hospital's stock. We have learned from the hit, but it would have been better to have learned from the near misses.

Interestingly, when the first batch of the new machines was delivered, the new model had a modification that looked as though it was specifically designed to prevent this very mishap. The controls were embedded in a steeply sloping surface, and any object placed there would slip off onto the floor. Did the manufacturers know something that we did not?

On the bright side, however, research into direct hits is beginning in medicine. In heart surgery as in many other surgical specialties, the boundaries of what can be successfully done, and to whom it can be done, are being constantly pushed back. Nowadays, patients are a lot older and a lot sicker than they were 20 years ago, and yet the overall results are better and the success rates are higher. Not surprisingly, the medical literature teems with reports of successful intervention in supposedly 'hopeless' cases.*

In the FIASCO study, (Freed 2009), my colleagues and I at Papworth took a diametrically opposite approach. Instead of looking at survivors of very high-risk surgery, we looked at those who died from very low-risk surgery. The reason for this was simple: we felt that the best way to identify any weaknesses in our care system was to take patients where nothing should have gone wrong and yet it did. We thought that, by analysing these cases, we could divide them into two groups. The first group would consist of those where death happened owing to 'a bolt from the blue' or 'an act of God': in other words, where death was a bit of bad luck that nobody could have foreseen or avoided. The second group would be those deaths that could have been foreseen and possibly prevented. It is in this second group that we believed we would find what went wrong that was avoidable, and, if a pattern emerged, we would know what needed to be fixed. The results were a real eye-opener.

We studied only those patients whose predicted mortality was less than 2 per cent, so they were low-risk patients who nobody expected would die. There were 4,294 such patients operated on between 1996 and 2005, and only 16 of them died, which gives a mortality of less than half a per cent, so that, on the face of it, we were, as a hospital, doing very well. We then meticulously reviewed the case notes of the 16 patients who died, and decided whether

---

*   Surgeons like nothing more than to publish papers with the unwritten subtitle 'Look how clever I am'.

the death was a 'freak', and therefore unavoidable, or whether it happened because of a FIASCO ('failure in achieving a satisfactory cardiac outcome'), and was therefore avoidable. Having thus classified the deaths, we sent the case notes to an independent outside expert to confirm that we had got the classification right. Both we and the independent outsider agreed that nine of the 16 deaths could not have been avoided, but that there were seven avoidable FIASCOs. A pattern emerged in which the two commonest reasons for death in this group were communication errors and an inadequate method of protecting the heart during the operation. Both have since been addressed at the hospital by a change of practice. Four years later, we carried out a follow-up study (FIASCO II) to see if these errors had been eliminated. The study showed that not a single patient in this period had died as result of communication errors or poor heart protection (Farid 2013). The lessons had been learned.

No heart operation is without risk. Mortality, though fortunately rare, can still occur, even in low-risk patients. Nevertheless, we were astounded to find that, even despite an extremely low mortality in the low-risk group, FIASCO still accounts for nearly a half of deaths. This suggests, even proves, that mortality may be reduced even further as part of a quality-improvement programme. All hospitals are different, and systemic weaknesses and strengths will not be the same in all of them. We therefore recommended that all hospitals do a FIASCO-type analysis on their own patients to see what can be fixed, if anything, in their systems. The first FIASCO paper was published some five years ago. At the time of writing, the grand total number of hospitals worldwide who took our recommendations and did their own analyses is, to the best of my knowledge, five: the Karolinska Hospital in Stockholm, Sweden, and a group of four hospitals in Turkey.

There is therefore still some ostrich-like behaviour among doctors and surgeons regarding the concepts of quality management, monitoring, and learning from mistakes. The overwhelming majority of doctors, surgeons included, and other healthcare workers are passionate about doing the best for their patients. The only problem is that there is an attitude of risk-taking, and a resistance to change. I alluded to this earlier as eminence-based medicine, which I defined as continuing to make the same mistake over and over again but with ever-increasing conviction. There is no doubt that at least some of this attitude persists in medicine. We are nowhere near the levels of self-examination and scrutiny that the aviation industry, and so many other fields of human endeavour, have already achieved, but there are signs that this is finally changing. Many hospitals now encourage incident reporting to see what can be learned from adverse events. Some even encourage near-miss reporting. In 2002, the Virginia Mason Hospital in the USA introduced 'Patient Safety Alerts', essentially a system for reporting anything that could potentially harm a patient. Take-up of the system by staff was muted at first, but, in 2004, a 69-year-old patient, Mrs Mary McClinton, died at the hospital as a result of an injection error, and this galvanised the staff into reporting near misses. As a result, the numbers of errors and medical accidents were drastically reduced, and the hospital benefited from a substantial reduction in its medical-liability insurance premiums. Elsewhere, near-miss and direct-hit reporting is also slowly increasing, though the systems designed to deal with both of these are still relatively rudimentary.

In *Better*, the American surgeon and writer Atul Gawande reveals how doctors can improve their services to patients in many walks of life, from the latest Western high-tech medicine to the provision of the most basic healthcare and vaccination programmes in remote villages in India. When the book was first published in 2007, I had the good fortune to be asked to review it for a medical journal, and I thoroughly enjoyed reading it. Here was someone who clearly had a longstanding and deep interest in the fields of safety, efficiency improvement, and error reduction in surgery. What's more, one of his ideas was to me an absolute revelation. He wrote that he realised that he could improve the care of his patients much more effectively not by finding new and cleverer things to do, but by continuing to do exactly what he already does, except doing it a little better.

In 2010, 817 people died in aeroplane crashes worldwide. In 2011, 17 American civilians died in terrorist attacks worldwide, which, incidentally, is about the same number as died by furniture falling on them. Between May 2010 and May 2012, nobody died of a terrorist attack in Britain. Now try to work out in your head the millions, if not billions, spent on aviation safety and terrorism prevention, and let us put cardiac surgery in context. About 39,000 major heart operations are carried out in the UK every year. The mortality is around 2 per cent, so that means around 780 patients die every year as a result of or after heart surgery.* This is the equivalent of two fully laden jumbo jets. Imagine the reaction of the media and the public to the loss of hundreds of lives if two jumbo jets crashed every year in the UK. Try to envisage the investigations, reports, mechanisms, safety measures, recommendations, and endless legislation that would follow such air-travel catastrophes.

Of course, we can expect there to be deaths in major surgery such as heart operations, and the death rate will never be zero.

---

* In Australia, with a similar mortality rate but a smaller population, the comparable figure is under 400 patients per year; in the US, the comparable figure is more than 6,000 patients per year.

Nevertheless, I hope that I have shown by now that simple steps can be taken to reduce this death rate, that some of these steps have been taken, that there is yet more to do, and that this a field where a little effort to do things a little bit better may well be richly rewarding for all of us.

6

Decisions, Decisions

Decades ago, patients pretty much did what doctors told them to do. The doctor, as expert, was trusted to know the right answer to a problem, and the patient, as a general rule, went along with the treatment prescribed by the expert. This is changing. The role of the passive patient has gradually shifted into that of an active consumer of health care. The catchphrase is 'No decision about me without me'. This is an understandable and legitimate shift. In making healthcare decisions, the patient makes a choice between no treatment and what can be an array of different available treatments, each with its own set of risks and benefits, and such decisions require information and intelligent process. In fact, whether a certain patient receives a certain treatment is perhaps the most important question that doctors and patients ever tackle. From the doctor's point of view, this is probably the one thing for which a medical education is essential. Pretty much everything else that is done by doctors and surgeons can be done by someone else with the right training.

Here are some of the things doctors do routinely: they take and record a medical history from patients, take blood samples, insert a catheter into the bladder, do an electrocardiogram, order a chest X-ray, prescribe medications, put up intravenous infusions, harvest veins from the leg for CABG, resuscitate a patient in cardiac arrest, and so on. Only 30 years ago, the mere idea of a non-doctor performing these duties would have been anathema to doctors and non-doctors alike. Nowadays, all of these tasks and more are performed by nurses and other healthcare professionals routinely and safely in many hospitals and in many parts of the world. The one thing that really, absolutely needs a full medical education is the thorny issue of selecting the right treatment for the disease, and offering it to the patient. In short, it is the decision-making. For that, doctors need a thorough education to make the right decisions, and patients need a reasonable level of knowledge to agree to or reject the treatment on offer. This is all the more important in surgery, as the consequences of the wrong decision (or the right decision that goes awry) can be disastrous. One day, you or a loved one will be faced with the offer of an operation. Deciding whether to accept that offer is not straightforward, but it can be done intelligently with a little understanding of the mechanisms necessary for decision-making. Before I explain the evidence-based way in which doctors go about this decision-making, we need to ask ourselves a simple yet crucially important question: why do doctors treat patients?

Why indeed? It is a question that I often put to my fourth-year medical students, and some of them get the answer right, but many get it wrong, so let's begin by clarifying why doctors should *not* treat patients.

Poor reasons for treating patients:

- the patient has a disease
- the doctor has a treatment

- the doctor needs money
- the doctor wants the patient to go away quickly
- the patient wants to go home with some form of treatment.

All of these are not good reasons to administer medical treatment. There are only two good reasons for a doctor to treat a patient, and they are:

- to improve symptoms (help the patient to feel better)
- to improve prognosis (help the patient to live longer).

Any medical treatment that does not achieve at least one or the other of the above objectives should absolutely not be offered to the patient, because this would be unethical. A treatment that neither improves symptoms nor improves prognosis is at best useless and at worst both dangerous and a costly waste of resources.

The only exception to the above rule is in the field of immunisation, where on occasion it can be justified to offer vaccinations against a particular disease to all people (even those who are not susceptible to the disease) in order to increase the 'herd immunity' and thus eradicate or drastically reduce the impact of a nasty disease. Even then, receiving the vaccination can often have prognostic benefit to the individual, so that the rule remains intact in most vaccination programmes.

Surgery is no exception. The reason, or 'indication', for an operation is always either symptomatic (to reduce or abolish troublesome symptoms, such as pain, discomfort, breathlessness, itching, palpitations, and so forth) or prognostic (to improve the likelihood of survival). In other words, the symptomatic indication deals with quality of life, and the prognostic indication deals with quantity of life.

So our original question naturally branches out into two parts:

- Is the operation the right choice to relieve the symptoms?
- Will the operation improve survival?

Let us deal first with the symptomatic indication, which is the simpler one of the two. In surgery (as opposed to general medicine), the symptomatic indication must fulfil an essential criterion that is always the same, regardless of the patient, the nature of the symptom, the surgical specialty, the surgeon in question, and the envisaged operation. It is a simple criterion that applies to all: there is no indication for surgery for symptoms until medical treatment has failed. The reason for this is obvious: patients in their right mind would never choose to have a hairy-armed surgeon cut them open with a knife if there is a tablet that achieves the same symptomatic relief. So the first question becomes: is the symptom successfully controlled by tablets? If the answer is 'Yes', keep taking the tablets. If the answer is 'No', consider surgery.

When medical treatment with tablets has failed, and surgery is being contemplated for symptoms, the next decision is whether to take the plunge and have the operation, and that is where risk comes into it. The patient must weigh up how troublesome the symptom is against the risk of the operation. For example, if a patient has angina, and the risk of a CABG to cure the angina, as calculated by a risk model (and perhaps adjusted to the surgeon's own performance) is a mortality of 1 per cent, the patient needs to decide if he or she is prepared to accept a risk to life of 1 per cent to get rid of the angina. This is a relatively easy decision to make:

the patient knows how troublesome the angina is, and its impact on quality of life, and most patients can easily understand what 1 per cent, or one in 100, means. The patient can therefore make an informed decision as to whether he or she thinks the benefit of the operation is worth the risk.

Deciding on having an operation for prognosis is much more problematic. On the face of it, nothing could be easier, as no symptoms are involved, only prognosis (survival) and risk. Because the operation is being contemplated for survival, we know that the condition or disease must carry a risk to life if not treated: in other words, not having the operation carries a risk. The operation itself also carries a risk. All we have to do is find out which risk is the smaller one, and, hey-presto, we have a decision.

Unfortunately, there is a catch.

The problem is that the risk of the operation is immediate, upfront, now. The risk of not having the operation is spread over time. If you have a condition that might kill you in the future, and you are thinking about having an operation to fix it tomorrow morning, you can be fairly certain that tomorrow night you are more likely to be alive if you do *not* have the operation. But you are not simply interested in tomorrow; you also care about next week, next month, and next year. You may also, depending on how young you are, be acutely interested in the next decade, or even the next 20 or 30 years. So how do you decide? And what information do you need to help you do so?

Let us assume that you are having a heart operation with a total risk to life of 5 per cent (3.5 per cent during the hospital stay, and another 1.5 per cent in the first three months after surgery), after which your survival becomes 'normal', in that it will follow the normal pattern for people of your age and sex, as shown by the graphs built from data used by insurance companies. The survival curve for a group of 100 patients just like you having surgery would look like this:

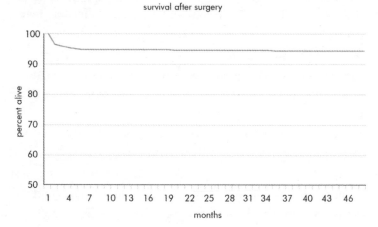

survival after surgery

There is a sharp dip immediately after the operation, and thereafter the curve levels off and follows the normal survival pattern for people without the disease.

Now let us assume that you have decided *not* to have the operation, and that the disease kills about 5 per cent of the patients who carry it every year. Your survival graph without an operation would look something like this:

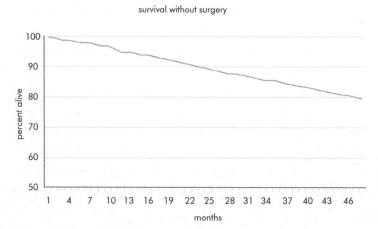

survival without surgery

To compare the two, we superimpose the graphs one on top of the other, and end up with something like this:

surgery versus no surgery

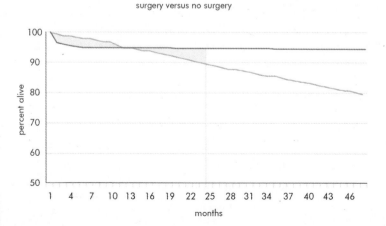

It is pretty obvious that, up to about a year, you would be more likely to be alive if you have *not* had an operation. In fact, at about a year, the same percentage of patients is alive in both groups, but more years of life have been lost in the group who opted for surgery. From about a year onwards, things change, and the ones who have chosen to have an operation begin to outlive those who chose not to have an operation. Now look at the next graph:

surgery versus no surgery

It is identical to the previous one, except that two areas between the lines have been shaded. These areas are equal in size, and they are the difference in years of life lost between those who had surgery and those who had not. When the lines cross, an equal number of people are alive in the two groups, but those who had surgery lost more years of life. At just over 24 months, the ones who did *not* have surgery have lost as many years of life as the ones who did, and, from then onwards, surgery can only be good for your survival. That point is crucial, and the length of time it takes you to reach it after an operation is called 'time until treatment equipoise', or TUTE for short (Noorani 2014). When TUTE takes place is a vital piece of information that can help doctors and patients decide whether or not to have an operation *purely for survival*. The range can be astounding. In heart conditions where an operation is carried out to improve survival alone, TUTE can range from a few hours to a few decades.

Remember, however, that most operations are still carried out for symptoms, and the decision in such a scenario is easy: do the symptoms bother you enough to justify the risk? If so, have it. If not, tell the surgeon to put away the scalpel and leave you alone. Increasingly these days, however, patients who feel fine are being offered surgery for prognosis. When that happens, they (and their doctors) should know what the TUTE is, because it can be very, very different from one patient to the next and from one condition to the next. For example, an otherwise healthy middle-aged man with a narrowing in the left coronary artery has a TUTE of only a few weeks for a CABG operation: if he opts for surgery, a few weeks down the line he is more likely to be alive than if he opts for no surgery, so that it is virtually a no-brainer that he should take the plunge. On the other hand, for an 85-year-old woman with an aneurysm of the aorta, the TUTE may well be six years or more:

that means it will be at least six years after the operation before she is more likely to be alive with than without surgery. Armed with knowledge, she may well politely decline the heroic surgeon's plan for fixing her aorta.

The TUTE concept is relatively new, but I have tested it on many patients from all backgrounds and all levels of educational attainment, and they all understood it perfectly. Of course, we cannot calculate TUTE unless we know for sure the risk of an operation and the natural history of the disease without an operation. These are not fully and exactly determined for all conditions and all operations, but we already have enough data in the medical literature to work things out for many conditions and procedures, and, as time passes, we will know more and more. I would like the TUTE method to be used in decision-making by both patients and doctors when operations are planned for the sole purpose of improving survival, and I believe that, one day, when we know with reasonable certainty the value of TUTE for all types of conditions, it may well be. When that is done, the TUTE concept may also be applied to quality of life. Many operations are designed to improve quality of life, but there is no doubt that, immediately after surgery, an operation worsens quality of life. After a major operation, the patient needs to recover from the surgery itself, get over the pain and complications, be rehabilitated, and return to normal life before beginning to benefit from the promised improvement in quality of life. TUTE in such a scenario is equally important, especially if the patient is elderly and not expected to live very long in the first place. There have, to date, been no studies whatsoever examining the net balance of quality-of-life benefits and disadvantages when major surgery is carried out in the elderly, but this will soon change.

7

The Trouble with Ratings

We have seen how surgeons can improve their mortality record by actually killing more patients. With a little expertise, manipulation, and perhaps some malice, a less good surgeon may be rated higher than a better one. Sadly, however, this is not the only reason why league tables can be misleading. They can mislead with no malice at all. All it takes is a little ignorance.

One of the few legacies that Margaret Thatcher's government left on the NHS was some degree of fiscal probity and accountability. She and her ministers were keen that hospitals did their accounts appropriately, were able to explain income and expenditure, and learned to budget properly. To some extent, this was successful. When Tony Blair's Labour government took office, it shifted the emphasis from pennies to outcomes, and wanted to measure how well hospitals were doing things. The Department of Health picked a handful of conditions, and asked hospitals to measure their outcomes for these conditions. One of them was heart attacks.

We have seen in Chapter Two that a heart attack occurs when a narrowed coronary artery gets completely blocked, usually by a fresh clot that forms on a furred-up area (or plaque) in the wall of artery. As the clot blocks the blood flow down the artery, the part of the heart muscle that this artery was feeding simply dies. The patient gets a terrible chest pain that doesn't get better with the usual measures. The heart may fail if the piece of muscle that dies is big enough. There may be dangerous disturbances in the rhythm of the heart, or the heart may stop completely. The bit of dead muscle may give way, causing a rupture with severe bleeding in the chest, or a hole may form in the heart, or a valve may give way and start to leak very badly. It all depends on where (and how big) the dead bit of heart muscle is. Not surprisingly, some of these complications can be fatal, and that is why people sometimes die from heart attacks. Most, fortunately, do not. They are admitted into a coronary care unit, where they receive treatment to prevent and manage all of these complications, and doctors try to reduce the size of any dead bit by re-opening the artery (if you can get at it fast enough).

Heart attacks are common, and survival is an objective and reasonable outcome for measuring how well they are treated, which is why the UK government was interested in them. So hospitals were ranked according to their individual heart attack mortality, and, in the interest of transparency, the results were made available to the public: a heart attack league table was born. My own hospital, Papworth, was the absolute worst, with a mortality of 40 per cent for heart attack, whereas most had a mortality of between 10 and 15 per cent. It was appalling news. Patients awaiting heart surgery were calling us in a panic, and the hospital management team thought that we had a real problem on our hands.

We began to wonder where this 40 per cent figure came from. Normally, at the time of this report, patients with heart attacks were admitted to acute general hospitals. These are hospitals with

Accident & Emergency departments equipped to deal with most emergencies, and having a coronary care unit specifically to admit patients with heart attacks. At the time of that league table, we were not an acute hospital, and we did not have a coronary care unit. In other words, we simply did not admit patients with acute heart attacks: they went to two other general hospitals nearby. A brief search into our data promptly revealed what was going on. The reason we had such a 'high mortality from heart attack' was not that we were bad, but that the only patients we treated with this condition were those who came to us *in extremis* from the two other nearby hospitals and from other general hospitals in our region.

Rarely, the part of the heart that dies in a heart attack is the muscle between the two pumping chambers, or ventricles, of the heart. Even more rarely, the dead muscle gives way, creating a defect or hole, with blood going round in circles within the heart and lungs instead of nourishing the body. The condition is called ventricular septal rupture. When that happens, the patient becomes very sick indeed, rapidly progressing into heart, lung, and kidney failure. Death is usually inevitable unless the defect is closed surgically. It is, of course, a very high-risk operation carried out urgently on a sick heart that has not yet recovered from the ravages of a big heart attack, so it is not surprising that it is an operation with very high mortality. Up to about half of the patients who have this operation die from it, but at least it offers some chance of survival, so it is better than doing nothing. When doctors in a coronary care unit in one of the hospitals around us make the diagnosis of ventricular septal rupture, they normally refer the patient to us for emergency surgery.

In the period covered by the heart attack league table, there were five such patients with ventricular septal rupture, and they were the only 'heart attack' patients we had treated. Two died: 40 per cent, which is actually a pretty good result. We managed, eventually, to re-assure our other patients and their relatives that they were, in fact, safe to be treated at our hospital, but the cost to us and to our patients of this 'transparency' was substantial.

We live in an age where transparency is a buzzword. Politicians and the media never tire of asking for more of the stuff. Predictably, their enthusiasm for transparency rapidly seems to fizzle out when they are asked to provide some clarity about their own, often sordid, affairs. Regardless of their behaviour, we lesser mortals providing public services are nowadays expected to provide a transparent insight into our work patterns and outcomes, and the field of healthcare is no exception. If those who work in healthcare generally are not immune from constant demands for more transparency, then those specialties in which good data are available are much more susceptible than others. After all, it is pretty difficult actually to demand open access to data from a specialty that does not collect any data. For that reason, my own specialty of cardiac surgery has found itself an easy target in the firing line of the 'more-transparency-now' big guns.

After the public outrage that followed the Bristol Royal Infirmary affair, heart surgeons found themselves in the unenviable position of having lost much of the public's confidence in them. One of the recommendations of the Bristol inquiry was to push hard for transparency and the publication of results, and the Department of Health at the time had made this issue a priority. Somewhat reluctantly, with many dissenters and loud interminable arguments at national specialty meetings, the cardiac surgical profession agreed to work towards the publication of outcomes, and this has now happened. If you go to www.scts.org and follow the links 'Patients' and 'Heart surgery in the UK', you will find web pages with access to the data from every heart surgery hospital in the country, with survival figures for overall heart surgery and certain specific operations, most of which will have been risk-adjusted using EuroSCORE or a more stringent version of EuroSCORE, and most hospitals will have provided data subdivided by individual consultant surgeons. You can, if you wish, scrutinise my own outcomes for heart surgery. In terms of transparency, heart surgery has already achieved much more than other areas of medicine, and the UK has achieved much more than other countries.

Yet the journey towards this level of transparency was not without pitfalls. On 1 January 2005, the Freedom of Information Act came into force in the UK. In grossly simplified terms, the act mandates that information collected by public bodies using publicly provided resources should be made available within 20 days to any member of the public who requests it. Shortly before the act became law, the chief executive of Papworth Hospital received a letter from *The Guardian* newspaper, informing him that it was the paper's intention to submit an official request under the act to provide the data on the hospital's mortality for coronary artery bypass grafting (CABG). He asked me what we should do, and the answer to my mind was obvious: we should, of course, comply. We had the data, we were proud of the data, and it was the law! A quick check with colleagues elsewhere in the country confirmed that the chief executives of their hospitals had also received a letter from the newspaper, and some were quite perturbed by this sudden demand.

The Guardian, however, did not ask about risk profiles, so we guessed that the plan was to publish a league table for CABG with no attention to risk. This would mean that the listed figures would be misleading if the purpose was to inform the public. As we have already seen, when the mortality for CABG is 2 per cent in hospital X but only 1 per cent in hospital Y, there can be three possible reasons for the difference:

Reason 1: the difference is due to chance.

Reason 2: the difference is due to a different case mix (hospital X operates on many high-risk patients, and hospital Y operates on low-risk patients).

Reason 3: hospital Y is better.

Before we can conclude that hospital Y is better than hospital X, we need to know the confidence intervals around the measurements (in other words, whether the difference is real or due to chance). Once that is established, we need to know the case mix of the patients (if the case mix in both hospitals is similar, hospital Y is truly better than hospital X). *The Guardian* had not asked for this information, and we felt that they should have asked, so we contacted them. Two days later, the two reporters working on this project came up from London to Cambridge to find out more. I explained to them the issues of statistical confidence and risk profiling, the use of risk models such as EuroSCORE, and the importance of taking account of these sorts of factors when reporting or publishing health outcomes. They took it all on board.

The article appeared on Wednesday 15 March 2005, as a front-page headline story backed by two whole pages in the main paper. The newspaper published the results for hospitals across the UK. Some were crude, some were risk-adjusted, and most were by hospital and surgeon. The data were divided into risk-adjusted and non-risk-adjusted, listed alphabetically, and with intelligent explanations about the results, the caveats needed in interpreting them, and the importance of statistical analysis and risk profiling. In other words, the paper behaved with integrity and responsibility, and avoided all temptation to sensationalise its findings.

Other newspapers have reported the same issues with far more lurid copy. If ten patients had died in one hospital and 30 in another, this would have been reported as 'SCORES OF PATIENTS ARE DYING NEEDLESSLY IN THE UK'. In the *British Medical Journal*, Dr Jan Poloniecki drew attention to other potential yet meaningless shock-horror headlines that could be paraphrased as 'HALF OF THE SURGEONS IN THE UK ARE BELOW AVERAGE'. This, of course, is absolutely true. It simply happens to be what the word 'average' means: half are above, and half are below. If they weren't, average wouldn't be average. Sensational and sloppy reporting of this nature can result in patients and the public getting the wrong message altogether, with unnecessary and distressing loss of confidence affecting perfectly competent, world-class health services. It is not, however, only the less savoury sections of the media that can thus mislead. Even the professionals can get it wrong.

Dr Foster is an organisation that took it upon itself to make hospital information available to the public. It is a professional outfit, with experts in both medicine and statistics on board. In the early days of its operation, it of course concentrated on cardiac surgery, presumably because the data were available and relatively easy to interpret, and the outcome measure (survival) was objective and obtainable. Dr Foster began to collect data by relying on information from Hospital Episode Statistics, or HES. This is a system in which clerks assign codes to patients when they leave the hospital. These codes include procedures performed on the patients during their hospital stay. Dr Foster thus identified from these data which patients had CABG and only CABG, and reported on the mortality. To this day, I vividly remember sitting, with fellow cardiac surgeons in the august hall of the Royal College of Surgeons in London to listen to eminent Dr Foster officials explain to us what data they had, how they acquired and analysed the data, and how they were going to make everything public in the interests of transparency.

HES data are notoriously inaccurate. The codes are chosen by poorly paid clerks, some of whom may not have had enough training in interpreting medical case notes. The medical case notes themselves are often incomplete. So I did not have a lot of confidence in the accuracy of whatever Dr Foster officials were going to tell us, but I nevertheless listened with an open mind. The spokesman said that they had taken great care in collating the data and ensuring that only CABG patients were included in their analysis. He assured the audience that Dr Foster were meticulous in identifying patients who had CABG plus 'something else', and took pains to exclude such patients from the data. 'Something else'? We had assumed that Dr Foster would remove patients who had CABG plus, say, a heart valve operation, or CABG plus replacement of the aorta, and so on. The spokesman went on to assure us that all of the patients who had CABG plus below-knee amputation were absolutely excluded from the analysis.

Excuse me? Below-knee amputation?

Now that is a most unusual combination, to say the least. The commonest isolated operation in cardiac surgery is CABG. The commonest combined operation is CABG plus replacement of the aortic valve. Of course, there are many other combinations of operations, but for a patient to walk into hospital one day and, a few days later, hobble out with a coronary artery bypass graft but minus a leg must be vanishingly rare. What was Dr Foster doing, looking at this category specifically to exclude it, and to re-assure us that it was excluded from analysis? From that point onwards, I stopped paying attention to the slick presentation on the podium, and my mind wandered as I was trying to figure out why on Earth a patient would come into hospital for a CABG and a leg amputation in the first place. Try as I might, I could not think of a credible clinical scenario. Then I remembered that Dr Foster studies HES data. These data record the codes for what actually happened during the hospital episode, rather than what the patient originally came into hospital for. Illumination finally dawned.

The confounding factor was a marvellous invention called the intra-aortic balloon pump, or IABP. This clever device is one of the few medical gadgets that could be described as a true lifesaver. It is a pump that helps the ailing heart, especially if the heart is being starved of blood supply and oxygen, because of narrowed arteries. The IABP can, in specialist units, be connected to the patient and activated in about 10 to 20 minutes at the bedside. The doctor puts a needle in the femoral artery, then threads a wire through the needle so that the wire comes up the femoral artery into the descending aorta, which courses along the spine. The wire stops when it reaches the top of the aorta, in the chest. Over this wire, a specially designed long sausage-shaped balloon is inserted so as to lie within the aorta, some 20 centimetres downstream of the heart. The balloon is connected to the pump, and the pump can read the patient's heart beat. When activated, the pump rapidly inflates the balloon with helium while the heart is relaxing, and rapidly sucks out the helium and flattens the balloon when the heart is pumping, so that it follows the action of the heart, but beats out-of-synch with it. This provides two huge advantages: the first is that, by deflating the balloon just as the heart is about to start pumping, it cuts down the pressure in the aorta, making the heart's job much easier (it is easier to pump blood into a low-pressure system than a high-pressure one). The second is that, by inflating and raising the blood pressure when the heart is relaxing, it forces blood down the coronary arteries, improving the blood supply to a heart that may be starved of oxygen. An IABP can get a patient out of heart failure better, quicker, and more effectively than any drug, and patients whose angina is so bad that they are teetering on the edge of a full-blown heart attack find the angina instantly relieved as they are pulled back from the brink by the IABP. One of the most satisfying procedures in medicine is setting up the IABP in an awake patient. The instant that the pump is switched on, the patient smiles, and thanks the doctor for getting rid of the angina pain.

Such a machine is a godsend to heart surgeons, especially those doing CABG on critical patients. If the heart is not working too well at the end of the operation, the IABP buys time, gives the heart a rest, and allows it to recover over the next couple of days. Yet in surgery, as in everything else, there is no such thing as a free lunch. IABPs have their complications, and one of those complications relates to the point at which the balloon is inserted, and where it stays during the course of the treatment: it is, of course, the femoral artery in the leg. If the femoral artery is damaged by the procedure, or bleeds, or fills up with clot, or is small and gets blocked by the sheer physical size of the balloon, then the leg is at risk. Very rarely, the leg is damaged beyond salvation, and a below-knee amputation is carried out.

That is why Dr Foster found the strange combination of below-knee amputation and CABG. These were standard CABG operations that went badly wrong, needed an IABP, which itself went badly wrong, and lost the hapless patient a leg. And what did Dr Foster want to do with these patients in their league tables? Why, exclude them of course, thinking they were not standard isolated CABG. Yet such patients absolutely must be included in any league table looking at the success and failure of CABG, because they are precisely the ones where things went horribly wrong. The problem was that the highly intelligent folk at Dr Foster simply did not know that.

Since that particular episode, Dr Foster have improved massively in their understanding of the data that they analyse and report, and I do not think that errors quite as glaring as this would happen today in their reporting. Nevertheless, this example illustrates yet another danger of publishing league tables when the data from which they are derived are not analysed intelligently.

Heart surgeons and their patients are now accustomed to the publication of outcomes, but other specialties are not. They will have to learn fast: on 28 June 2013, the NHS began publishing the outcomes of surgery in a non-cardiac surgical specialty. For the first time ever, the results of vascular surgery (surgery on blood vessels) were being made available in the public domain, and those of other surgical specialties will follow. Many of these non-cardiac surgical specialties do not, as yet, have sophisticated risk-assessment models, and the data are therefore even more likely to be misread and misinterpreted than in heart surgery. Transparency is, of course, a good thing, and league tables of results may indeed inform the public about the outcomes of healthcare, so that an individual patient and his or her family can make an informed choice, but there are many, many dangers for the unwary.

I have shown some examples where reported numbers can be meaningless without appropriate statistical analysis, and other examples where comparisons can mislead and even cause panic because they are not comparing things that are comparable. I have also shown how a bad surgeon can look better than a good surgeon in a league table, and given some examples where vital data can be missed out altogether in the analysis so that entire league tables are misleading. Finally, I hope to have convinced you that patients and doctors alike can be damaged by irresponsible and half-baked sensationalist reporting by those sections of the media keener on headlines and profit than on truth.

That, unfortunately, is not all.

The greatest risk to the patient in the publication of league tables is that the surgeons start to run away from high-risk surgery, and that is bad news indeed, especially if you are such a patient.

The coronary artery bypass graft operation is probably the most studied, scrutinised, researched, and reported therapeutic intervention in the history of medicine. Compared with most therapies, our knowledge about CABG is truly massive. We know who will benefit in terms of relief of symptoms. We know who is likely to live longer as a result of CABG, and who is likely to die if not offered a CABG. We know the likely risk of the operation to a relatively high degree of precision, and can tailor a custom-made quote for each individual patient having it. We also know the risk of *not* having CABG, and can compare the two. We have a pretty good idea of how long a CABG will last, and which of your three bypasses in a triple CABG will probably continue to function right up to the day you die of something else, such as being run over by a bus.

We also know that patients with weak hearts are more likely to die if they get a CABG than patients with strong hearts, but, despite that, other things being equal, patients with weak hearts should be even keener to go under the knife and receive a CABG. The reason for this is simple: if CABG is a little riskier for the weak-hearted, then not having a CABG is much, much worse. This has often been called the cardiac surgical paradox, and it can be stated simply, and brutally, like this: the more the operation is likely to kill you, the better it is for you.

This strange maxim does not simply apply to CABG, but also to many other areas of heart surgery. It sounds paradoxical, yet it is fairly easy to understand why it is true. By and large, simple operations done for simple things in the heart are low-risk, but so are the conditions that they treat, whereas complex, horrendous operations are done for complex, horrendous conditions, and these conditions are more likely to kill if left untreated. Recall the somewhat extreme condition of ventricular septal rupture. It is almost 100 per cent fatal if untreated, with a 40–50 per cent mortality rate if treated. Which would you rather have?

That brings us to the problem. Let us imagine a typical heart surgeon. He is now subject to transparency and close scrutiny, and his results are published on the web for all to see. He is on call one weekend when he is asked to see an 80-year-old female patient with a tired, weak heart. She has just had a heart attack, and had such bad angina afterwards that she had to be connected to an IABP. He looks at the results of her tests and sees that she has critical coronary disease, of the kind that leads rapidly to death without a CABG operation. He also sees that, after a long history of smoking and bronchitis, her lungs are not too great. The blood tests show that her kidneys are a tad dodgy as well. More worryingly, though, she is having chest pain despite being in bed, and even despite the medication and the IABP, meaning that she truly is on the brink of another heart attack, which will probably be fatal, so his only choice, if he is to do anything, is to operate now, as an emergency.

Being an educated and cautious surgeon, he calculates the risk of surgery using EuroSCORE II, the latest version of the risk calculator, and it tells him that the risk of her dying from surgery is 38 per cent. Without surgery, however, there is no way out for the patient. She will probably die from a heart attack soon, and even immediately if the IABP, which has kept her hanging on to dear life so far, is removed.

Our surgeon, however, is feeling rather good about himself. He has had a pretty good run so far. It is 27 March, four days before the end of the British financial year, in which he has done 72 CABG operations without a single death. His figures for this year will look amazing in the league tables. If he operates and she dies, his mortality jumps from zero to 1.4 per cent, which is roughly the national average. He is now faced with a dilemma. Surgery might be good for the patient, but may be bad for him, his figures, his private practice, and his naturally large ego.

Do league tables really deter surgeons from accepting high-risk patients? I recently surveyed the cardiac surgeons in the UK to find out. I asked them two simple questions. The questions, and the answers given by the cardiac surgeons, are given below:

A high-risk operation may be beneficial to a particular patient. Despite this, a cardiac surgeon may decide not to offer that option to the patient, and recommends continuing medical treatment. This is partly or wholly because of concern about the impact on that surgeon's figures should the patient opt for surgery and then succumb. Have you ever done this?

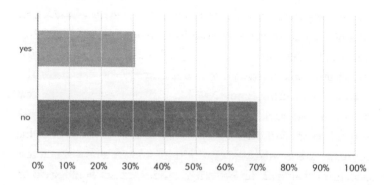

Are you aware of other surgeons doing this?

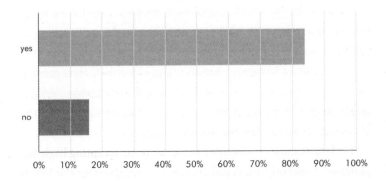

Of the 115 surgeons who responded to the survey questions, 35 (just under a third) admitted to denying surgery to patients who may benefit because of concern about their figures, and the great majority (84 per cent) reported that they were aware of other surgeons doing the same thing.

This survey has confirmed without any doubt that the clinical decision-making process of surgeons has indeed been adversely affected by the culture of transparency. Most surgeons who responded to the survey reported that they had seen such risk-averse behaviour in their colleagues, and nearly a third were honest enough to have reported such behaviour in themselves. The best interests of the patient, which should always come first, have had to take second place to the league tables.

With a health economist's hat on, one could argue that healthcare systems should probably not be offering high-risk surgery to anyone. The fact that such surgery is expensive, that resources are limited, and that the risk makes the operation less beneficial than in a young, otherwise fit person would seem to back this view, but we are forgetting two important considerations when we follow such a train of thought. The first is that doctors are primarily here to do the best for their patients (and not for the healthcare budget or their league-table figures). The second is the cardiac surgical paradox: the more an operation is likely to kill you, the better it is for you. This is simply because, in many such patients, withholding an operation has such a dismal outcome that the risk is more than amply justified. Yet withholding an operation and similar risk-averse behaviour unfortunately happens all too frequently. It is another reason why we should approach league tables with great care and circumspection. Sometimes, the price of transparency is unacceptable. Our poor old patient, if she is refused an operation, will die and become a statistic, but not a statistic that appears in the league table of heart surgery, and nobody will ever know.

Transparency is here to stay, and nothing we can do will turn the clock back. We can mitigate some of its damage by ensuring that the data are as accurate as possible, that all published data are properly adjusted for risk, that the analysis is statistically sound, and that the data are presented intelligently, but no matter what we do, we can never get away from the fact that, for a surgeon, the easiest and most effective way to reduce mortality is to say 'No' to high-risk patients, that the temptation to do so is a strong one, and that many surgeons will yield to it. There are, however, two things we can do. The first is to introduce a structure that allows surgeons to take on very high-risk patients without fear of damaging their own career and professional status, as illustrated by something called the Star Chamber.

When it comes to operating on very high-risk patients, the following facts are apposite. First, the cardiac surgical paradox often means that the patient, provided he or she survives, will stand to benefit enormously from the operation, and, if an operation is not carried out, the outlook is pretty bleak. Second, the surgeon, if the patient survives, will get kudos and feel good, but if the patient dies, will suffer physically, psychologically, and professionally. For a surgeon with even the tiniest scintilla of humanity, few things are worse than losing a patient. I know how I feel about it when it happens, and I have spoken at length about it to friends and colleagues. We all deal with the aftermath in different ways, but one feature of such a loss is common to all of us, and that is an overwhelming feeling of desperate loneliness. After all, the buck stops nowhere else but at our very door, if you will forgive the mixed metaphor. Third, in any particular group of surgeons, it tends to be the same ones who will take on the very high-risk patient, and who therefore have to take the 'hit' for everyone else if the patient dies. All of these are problems, but they can be turned into an opportunity.

At Papworth, we have always tended towards being one of those hospitals that accepts patients at the high end of the risk spectrum. National figures show that our patients are the oldest and have the sickest hearts in the country, and these differences are statistically significant. Even if we compare our patients with those of the hospital that accepts the second most elderly and sick patients, we also find the difference to be statistically significant. In other words, compared to the rest of the country, when it comes to how sick and high-risk the patients are, we are out on a limb: a true outlier.

As the culture of transparency and league tables began to take hold in cardiac surgery, our local motley crew of surgeons started to experience a certain feeling of unease about our particular type of high-risk practice, and this unease lay at the fork of a dilemma. We could proceed in one of two ways.

We could carry on in our merry way to take all comers,

regardless of risk, if we felt we could do them some good, but that would lay us open to ostracism should some of us begin to look bad in the league tables of surgeons. Even within Papworth, it tends to be a select group of us who are inclined to take on the very highest risk patients, and this is due to a combination of experience, specialised skills in certain operations, a pronounced desire to do the best for the patient regardless of risk, and, let's face it, sheer bloody-minded arrogance and self-confidence. When that is taken into consideration, we can see that this particular handful of surgeons would suffer more ostracism than most.

The alternative approach would be for us collectively to begin to say 'No' to the highest risk patients, like so many other surgeons and hospitals do already. The problem with this approach is that it would mean denying patients what could be their only chance, the loss of our hard-earned reputation as the hospital where 'anything is possible', and, last but not least, a serious dent to our collective professional ego.

That is when we came up with the concept of the Star Chamber. We never called it that. In fact, it went by the more prosaic title of the Surgical Council, and that is still its official title, but while I was explaining the concept to Bruce Rosengard, an American surgeon who worked at Papworth briefly, he exclaimed, 'Holy cow, you mean like a Star Chamber?', and the unofficial title stuck fast.

The original Star Chamber was an English court of law that sat at the royal Palace of Westminster from the 15th to the 17th century. Its intended purpose was to enforce the law against prominent, rich, and powerful people, who appeared immune to the efforts of the ordinary courts. The court of the Star Chamber sat in secret, with no indictments, no witnesses, no juries, and no right of appeal, and dispensed justice the way it saw fit. The court eventually became a somewhat dubious political weapon, used and abused by the monarchy. The idea formed the basis of a 1983 Hollywood film, also called *The Star Chamber* and set in modern times. In the movie, an idealistic vigilante judge finds ways of dispensing rough justice to any criminals who, in the view of the court, are guilty yet manage to escape punishment on a technicality. In the film version, the Star Chamber dispatches a hired killer to mete out capital punishment to those it finds guilty.

Needless to say, our Star Chamber did none of this, and its aim was certainly not to kill folk, but to offer an operation to those who would be at risk of being turned down by surgeons who are looking over their own shoulders at the league tables. It works very simply: any surgeon who is referred a patient considered to be at exceptionally high risk is encouraged to use the option of calling a meeting of the Star Chamber. Such patients may include those turned down by other hospitals, or those with a very high EuroSCORE (25 per cent or above), or any patient that the surgeon feels is exceptional in presenting a very difficult and high-risk challenge. The Chamber consists of all the consultant surgeons, but needs a minimum of four surgeons to attend in order to be quorate. The patient's case is then discussed in detail, and the Chamber makes three decisions: whether or not to offer surgery, the nature and strategy of the operation, and who in the group is best placed to do it, with the proviso that two consultant surgeons will be involved. This pair will perform the operation on behalf of the group, and the group will collectively take the full responsibility for the outcome.

On the face of it, the advantages of such an approach are legion. First, patients who would benefit from an operation will actually get their chance. Second, one would hope that the pair of surgeons who are best at this particular type of operation would be the ones selected to do it. Third, those selected to do it are working in the name of the group, and do not have to worry about their figures. And finally, the input of a group is always useful for covering all the bases (four heads being better than one), and that could mean a wiser, safer, and more carefully planned operation.

So far, the Star Chamber experiment has been a qualified success. On the positive side, many patients have been assessed through the system, and over half were offered operations, and most of these were successful. On the negative side, I feel sure that not all patients who are suitable have benefited from the approach, so that there may be some who were turned down without being considered, and others who were accepted by individual surgeons without consulting the Star Chamber. Interestingly, patients referred from elsewhere to the Star Chamber tended to do very well, whereas those brought by Papworth's own surgeons did less well, showing that it really takes a lot for a Papworth surgeon to be sufficiently frightened by a patient's level of risk to come to the Chamber.

Nevertheless, the Star Chamber continues to run at Papworth Hospital, providing a valuable service to some of the sickest heart patients in the country.

The second solution to the problems of risk-avoiding behaviour is to shift the emphasis in quality control from transparency onto a different, more robust and less harmful system.

Transparency means that outcomes are made public. It does not necessarily mean that they should be presented as a league table. *The Guardian* newspaper, for instance, was able to report all the data obtained from UK heart hospitals under the Freedom of Information Act without once succumbing to the temptation of presenting the results as a league table. On the contrary, the results were reported by hospital in alphabetical order, with separate subsections for those that used a risk-scoring method and those that did not. Other newspapers and sections of the media may not be so responsible, and the sensationalist lure of the hit parade is difficult to resist for an editor and a headline writer hungry for sales.

Let us pretend that you are a patient contemplating having a CABG somewhere in the UK, and you are presented with the following:

Institution	CABG Mortality
St Elsewhere Hospital	0.9%
Holby General Infirmary	1.2%
The Shire University Hospital	1.5%
The Heart Clinic	1.9%
Ambridge Royal Hospital	2.3%

Ambridge Surgeons	
Dr Green	1.8%
Dr Turquoise	2.1%
Dr Purple	2.4%
Dr Brown	2.7%

How likely is it that you will choose Ambridge Royal Hospital? And how likely is it that you will choose Dr Brown? Probably not at all likely. Yet Dr Brown and Ambridge Royal may well be statistically no better or worse than anyone else. They may even operate on higher-risk patients, and their results may actually be among the best in the country when the risk profile of their patients is taken into account. Nevertheless, I suspect most patients would run a mile if they saw the positions of Dr Brown and Ambridge Royal in the league table.

Let us now add to this toxic cocktail of potential misinformation a small dash of sensationalism: a newspaper reports the league tables not as an exercise in information and transparency, but as a shock-horror story, so that the front page is plastered with pictures of Dr Brown, carefully and deliberately chosen to make him look mean and unfriendly, along with an insert photograph of his suburban mansion on the outskirts of Borchester, with the inevitable million-pound price tag, another picture of his Porsche with its personalised number plate, and a headline screaming 'IS THIS THE WORST SURGEON IN BRITAIN?'

Apart from the inherent potential of misleading the public, league tables carry the substantial risk of putting whoever is the hapless surgeon or unfortunate hospital at the bottom of the league out of business altogether, so that if a newspaper publishes an account similar to the above, a surgeon's career may come to an end. When that happens, the surgeon stops appearing in the league table. Now that Dr Brown has gone, attention will focus on Dr Purple, who is now 'the worst surgeon in Britain', and the same will happen again. Taken to its logical conclusion, this process will eventually leave only one surgeon operating in the country. This is patently absurd. What is important for patients and their loved ones is not necessarily to have the 'best' surgeon in the 'best' hospital, but to know that the local hospital and surgeon that treat them by providing surgery are of a high standard that is considered up to scratch by modern criteria. In short, the patient needs and deserves an absolute guarantee that the surgical service treating him or her is one of quality. To that end, what we need is a system of quality accreditation.

The principle of quality accreditation is a very simple one. Hospitals should have in place a robust structure that ensures the following:

- The hospital knows what it does (numbers and types of operations).

- The hospital knows what the outcomes of these operations *should be* (this can be easily done by using a risk model).
- The hospital knows what its actual outcomes *are*.
- The hospital is satisfied that its outcomes are as they should be (by comparing them to the model).
- The hospital has a clear and well-established plan of action to be put into place immediately if it finds that its outcomes are not as they should be.

Now, these five requirements are not rocket science. They are easily within the capability of all hospitals doing surgery, and all they require is some rudimentary data collection and a little bit of paperwork. Indeed, I have argued that if you can't tell that your outcomes are up to scratch, you have no business doing heart surgery, or any other kind of surgery.

The European Association for Cardio-Thoracic Surgery, the European Society of Thoracic Surgeons, and the European Society for CardioVascular Surgery are the three biggest speciality societies in the fields of heart, lung, and vascular (blood-vessel) surgery in Europe. Some ten years ago, the three got together and established a body called ECTSIA, the European Cardiovascular and Thoracic Surgery Institute of Accreditation, which was empowered with offering official certificates of accreditation along the above lines to hospitals that were proven to satisfy these modest criteria and wanted their achievement recognised. To date, in all of Europe, the total number of hospitals that have applied and succeeded in obtaining this accreditation amounts to the grand sum of … three!

Perhaps many hospitals satisfy the criteria, but did not take the steps to achieve official recognition. Perhaps the initiative was not advertised widely enough, but this is unlikely to be the reason: I happen to know that when this quality accreditation plan was announced, no fewer than 500 different hospitals in Europe enquired about it and expressed an interest. From 500 to three is a huge drop. Could it be that even these simple structures are still not well developed enough for hospitals to take the plunge?

Building a system of proper quality accreditation of the type described above is a lot less 'sexy' than the transparency culture of publishing results, and attracts very little media interest, but it can ensure that robust quality-assurance and monitoring mechanisms are integrally woven into the very fabric of the way a hospital functions, and it can provide all patients with the peace of mind that comes with the knowledge that their surgery providers meet the acceptable standard. To use the American cliché, what's not to like?

8

Curious Influences

What is the oldest profession in the world? The stock answer is, as we all know, prostitution. However, a very long time before any prostitute ever walked the streets, and well before any female even existed, going right back to the genesis of the world in the Old Testament, we know that the Lord God '... took one of the man's ribs and then closed up the place with flesh' (Genesis 2:21–24). This, of course, was the famous rib from which Adam's companion, Eve, was supposed to have been made. Be that as it may, to us cardiothoracic surgeons, a rib resection is a rib resection, and it is a stock-standard operation in the surgical repertoire of any of us. This means that the world's oldest profession is, in fact, cardiothoracic surgery, and its first practitioner was God himself.

I used to enjoy telling this somewhat lame joke to anyone who would listen at medical dinners, until I was challenged by a particularly irritating anaesthetist who gleefully pointed out that the full text of that excerpt from Genesis is as follows (my italics):

So the Lord God *caused the man to fall into a deep sleep*; and while he was sleeping, he took one of the man's ribs and then closed up the place with flesh. Then the Lord God made a woman from the rib he had taken out of the man, and he brought her to the man.

In other words, the world's oldest profession was in fact not cardiothoracic surgery, but cardiothoracic anaesthesia.

There is little love lost between surgeons and anaesthetists. They work in close proximity to one another. They are separated only by a surgical drape. On one side of the drape is the anaesthetist, with the requisite paraphernalia of respiratory machines, monitoring equipment, and powerful drugs and the means to administer them. On the other side is the sterile field, the open wound, the blood, the sharp instruments, and the surgeon. This drape has been christened by some witty anaesthetist with the provocative name of the blood–brain barrier.* So to anaesthetists, they are the brain (intelligent, reasonable, thoughtful) and we surgeons are the blood (gory, impetuous, sanguine).

In the eyes of many surgeons, anaesthetists are lazy, crossword-obsessed tea and coffee addicts who would go to any length to avoid doing some work and who are constantly watching the clock, their only interest in the life-or-death operation taking place before their very eyes being summarised thus: 'When will this bloody procedure finish so I can go home?' Predictably, the view from the anaesthetic side of the blood–brain barrier is that surgeons are a bunch of bloodthirsty, arrogant, aggressive, overconfident

---

* There is a real blood–brain barrier: it is the intricate cellular and molecular complex that protects the brain by stopping certain drugs and other bad substances from crossing into the brain from the bloodstream, and has nothing to do with surgical drapes.

cowboys with massive egos and small brains. These are, of course, somewhat extreme caricatures, but, like all caricatures, there is more than just a grain of truth in them.

Anaesthetists can be viciously eloquent in mocking surgeons. In the second edition of the serious educational textbook *Core Topics in Cardiac Anaesthesia* by Jonathan Mackay and Joseph Arrowsmith, there is an appendix that contains a table of the phonetic alphabet. Alongside this, another table contains what the editors (both anaesthetists) describe as the 'surgical alphabet'. The phonetic alphabet of course goes like this:

Alpha, Bravo, Charlie, Delta, Echo, Foxtrot … and so on.

The surgical alphabet, according to McKay and Arrowsmith, goes like this:

Accuse, Blame, Criticise, Deny … and so forth.

Another famous and oft-repeated anaesthetic quip is that there are only two types of surgeons: the bastards and the slow bastards. A third is the very well-known 'definition' of anaesthesia:

Anaesthesia is the half-awake
watching the half-asleep
being half-murdered
by the half-witted.

There are many other examples of anaesthetic scurrilous attacks on surgeons, but it most certainly is not one-way traffic. If we surgeons have not yet quite reached the same exalted level of vitriolic invective in abusing our beloved anaesthetic colleagues, it certainly has not been for lack of trying:

You can easily identify the professions of those who work in an operating room by the spillage on their shoes: On the shoes of a cardiac surgeon, there is blood. On the shoes of a urologist, there is urine. On the shoes of a liver surgeon, there is bile, and on the shoes of a colorectal surgeon, there is, of course, shit. How do you recognise an anaesthetist? Easy: on their shoes, there's coffee.

One saying that is a favourite plaint by cardiac surgeons is the following:

Heart surgery is a team effort
(*until the patient dies, then it's just the surgeon's fault*)

This speaks volumes, if only to highlight how exasperated some surgeons are with the inescapable fact that they, and they alone, tend to be the ones held responsible for poor results, when the care is actually delivered by an entire team. Most people do not know that, in a standard cardiac operation such as CABG, there are, on average, around nine people working within the operating theatre, and they are as follows:

On the surgical side:

- the principal surgeon (conducting the operation)
- the assistant surgeon (helping the principal surgeon)
- the second-site surgeon (taking veins from the leg or elsewhere to use for constructing the coronary bypass)
- the scrub nurse (managing the instruments and helping all three surgeons).

The above members of staff are scrubbed, gowned, and gloved. The others, who are not scrubbed (and who are stationed beyond the blood–brain barrier), are:

- the 'runner' (nurse or practitioner delivering items to the scrub nurse, dealing with messages, and adjusting machinery)
- the anaesthetist (putting the patient to sleep; keeping the patient asleep, pain-free, and alive; and managing the vital signs and any drugs that are needed)
- the assistant to the anaesthetist (either a junior anaesthetist or another 'runner')
- the perfusionist (technical person running the heart–lung machine)
- the assistant to the perfusionist.

In total, then, with nine people working as a team to deliver an effective and safe operation, why is it that, if the patient dies, it is purely the surgeon's fault?

A few years ago, at the major annual national meeting of cardiothoracic surgeons in the UK, there was an important presentation dealing with the outcomes of surgery. Numbers of operations were presented, and so were their outcomes, and the distribution of such activity among all the heart surgery hospitals in the country. The hall was packed with surgeons from all over the nation as these results were presented, but this happens every year at this particular meeting. The novelty in this particular year was the announcement that these outcomes were now to be made public and presented alongside surgeons' names. Needless to say, not all the surgeons in the auditorium were especially thrilled with this idea. One particularly aggravated heart surgeon stood up and addressed the conference, saying that, in his opinion, when it came to death from heart surgery, the heart surgeon is merely an 'innocent bystander', or, put in other words, the death is everybody else's fault.

Many laughed at this somewhat polarised view, but the reality is that we were somewhere between two extremes. At one end, there was an increasingly prevalent culture that blamed the surgeon squarely and entirely for the outcome, and, at the other end, a minority represented by our surgeon who felt that a bad outcome was not at all his fault, but everybody else's. The truth, as always, probably lies somewhere in between. On listening to this exchange, a number of thoughts coursed through my mind. The first, I'm afraid, was a rather vicious one: I wondered whether that very same surgeon who claimed that he was merely an 'innocent bystander' when a patient dies would also rush to claim that he was merely an 'innocent bystander' when a brilliant and difficult operation goes particularly well, and the patient survives against the odds. Being of a somewhat uncharitable disposition, and knowing surgeons as well as I do, I thought 'Probably not'.

My second thought was a little more productive. We all know that the surgeon makes a difference to the outcome, but do other members of the team? Perhaps we should investigate this to find out. Which member of the team shall we investigate first? The answer, of course, came by itself, screaming loudly from all the rooftops through a megaphone: the anaesthetist! Who else?

Briefly, we looked at more than 18,000 patients operated on at Papworth Hospital up to the year 2012, with 21 senior surgeons and 29 senior anaesthetists in charge of conducting the operations. We examined their predicted mortality and their actual mortality, and tried to see if there was any evidence of significant variation associated with who the surgeon was, and also if there was any evidence of significant variation associated with who the anaesthetist was (Papachristophi 2014). What we found was extraordinary: who the surgeon was actually did make a difference. Who the anaesthetist was made not an iota of difference: there was no appreciable difference in outcomes that could be linked to the anaesthetist. In fact, we have just extended and further analysed the data on surgeons and anaesthetists, and actually measured their impact on survival. If you have a heart operation at Papworth Hospital, whether you survive or succumb to the operation will depend on the following factors: 97 per cent of the outcome is determined by EuroSCORE, just under 3 per cent is determined by which surgeon operates on you, and a measly 0.01 per cent depends on which anaesthetist puts you to sleep. To put it another way, by far the most important factor is you, your operation, and your risk factors. Which surgeon you choose has a minuscule effect, and it doesn't matter a jot which anaesthetist you have, so just go for the one with a friendly smile.

This study, published in the *Journal of Cardiothoracic and Vascular Anesthesia* in 2014, was important for two reasons. The first was that it confirmed that our anaesthetic department, which usually follows harmonious and standardised protocols, and administers anaesthetic care according to fairly rigid, pre-agreed guidelines, was safe no matter who the anaesthetist was. Other anaesthetic departments in other institutions do not necessarily do this, and various anaesthetists in other hospitals are free to select the methods of anaesthesia that suit them, their habits, and their prejudices. To my mind, this study provides a strong stimulus for similar studies to be conducted in such hospitals. If their findings are the same as ours, and there is no variation, then there is no problem, but, if they find that one anaesthetist has better outcomes than another, then there may be a strong case for studying the technique used by that anaesthetist to see if others could learn by adopting it and thus improve their results. My anaesthetist colleague Andrew Klein has just completed a similar study of a number of UK hospitals, and found that there is indeed variation in anaesthetic outcomes in some of them, and, in one of these hospitals, the effect of the anaesthetists has almost the same magnitude as the effect of the surgeon at Papworth. This study is not yet published, but, when it is, it will have important implications for the anaesthetic protocols (or lack of them) in some of these institutions.

The second reason was more personal. For the first time ever, I was able to give lectures to prominent anaesthetists in many parts of the world to show that we were unable to find that the anaesthetist had a discernible influence on outcomes, and conclude perfectly legitimately that, according to our study, we had proved that there is no such thing as a good anaesthetist.

You may well think that this is a little contrived, slightly petty, or frankly pathetic, but at least it scores one point for the surgeons in the endless and unequal war of abuse between these two great but disparate professions.

What about other external influences on the outcome of an operation? What can our quality-measurement tools reveal about those?

Arthur Hailey was a British-Canadian novelist who wrote a string of best-selling novels that almost always have an industrial or commercial backdrop. Among his most famous titles are *Hotel*, which became a successful and long-running television series; *Airport*, which was made into a Hollywood blockbuster; *Wheels*, which took in the American motor industry in Detroit; and *The Final Diagnosis*, which is set in a hospital pathology department, and happens to be my favourite. Hailey spent a very long time in the environments in which he set his novels, and his work is characterised by meticulous research and insider knowledge of the background to his stories. This meant that the casual reader effortlessly learned a massive amount about the intricacies of airports, hotels, and pathology departments while being entertained with multiple parallel storylines. As each strand seemed always to end a chapter on a cliffhanger, and the next chapter took up the cliffhanger from a previous strand, this had the effect of making the book truly difficult to put down despite the lamentations of the critics about the lack of literary style.

In *Wheels*, published in 1971, Hailey writes that a well-known fact in the motor trade is that one should avoid buying a car built on a Monday or a Friday. The reasons he gives for this are obvious and intuitive: on a Monday, the workers are dragging their feet back into the factory, and, on a Friday, they can't wait to get away, so that on both of these days their workmanship may be expected to suffer. I am not aware if any independent research has ever confirmed or refuted this allegation, but, as I have an obsession with the subject of the quality of surgical work, I could not help wondering whether surgeons may also be prone to such vagaries. I was not specifically interested in the Monday/Friday business, as surgeons, by and large, enjoy their work, and many of their long-suffering families would testify to the fact that it is difficult to get them to drag their feet away from the darned hospital rather than the other way around. What I wondered about, however, was the impact of a prolonged break, such as a holiday, or a prolonged period at work, such as on the day immediately before a holiday, on surgical performance.

It is conceivable that surgical skills need to be exercised continuously to be maintained, and that a holiday may cause these skills to become a little rusty, so having an adverse effect on performance on the first day back. It is also conceivable that the day immediately before a holiday is the last day of a prolonged work period without a break, and a surgeon may be tired or even feel burnt out, badly in need of a refreshing change and a rest, and perform sub-optimally as a result of these feelings. When you think about it, both scenarios are equally and unpleasantly plausible ones. With risk-adjusted outcomes readily available to us, it was not too difficult to find the answer (White 2007).

We studied 7,873 patients who had heart operations at Papworth Hospital over a four-year period, and we began by dividing these patients into three groups. The first group consisted of those patients who had their operations done on the very last day before a surgeon went on holiday. The second included those patients who had their operation on the very first day of the surgeon returning to work after a holiday. The third group (the majority) was the control group: everybody else. We adjusted all of these for risk, just in case one of the groups contained higher-risk patients than others, and we looked to see if mortality in the groups operated just before a holiday or just after a holiday differed from the rest. The results of this study were quite a revelation.

The first thing we found was that the patients were remarkably similar: our surgeons had clearly not made any special efforts to operate on (or to avoid operating on) particular types of patient if they were about to go on holiday, or if they had just come back: they took all patients as they came.

The second thing we found was that mortality for the entire group was only 4 per cent. For the period of the study at the beginning of the last decade, this was a good result overall. The mortality for the control group was similar to the total, but mortality in patients operated just before a holiday was more than double the mortality on the first day after a holiday. This did not quite reach statistical significance,* but there was a strong and persuasive trend.

---

* The p-value was 0.053. You need a p-value of less than 0.05 for the difference to be considered statistically significant.

The study confirmed irrefutably that holidays do not cause surgical skills to become rusty. On the contrary, there seemed to be a patient-protective effect of operating on the first day after an absence, and a patient-damaging effect of operating on the last day before hopping on the plane.

Why is that? There can be many reasons for this, but I have a theory relating to personality types that I will explain later on. In the meantime, surgeons who are planning a holiday would be well advised to stay at their desk on the last working day before the holiday, where they are likely to do less damage.

Another question that our new tools can address is whether surgeons should stop operating if a patient dies on the table. When a patient dies under the care of a physician rather than a surgeon, it is often the patient who gets the blame, and the stock phrase used is: 'I am sorry, but he or she "failed" to respond to the treatment.' The underlying assumption behind this platitude is that it was somehow the poor patient's fault. Of course, the right treatment will sometimes truly fail, and patients will sometimes fail to respond, or the wrong treatment is given, or the right treatment is given but badly, or there is no right treatment available. Any of these can and do cause treatment failure and death, but when a physician's patient dies while undergoing treatment, no automatic assumption is made that the physician prescribing the treatment is responsible.

This is somewhat different in surgery. When a patient is operated as an emergency with a view to salvage life, the surgeon may be treated in a similarly charitable and forgiving manner, and thus the patient may also be seen to have 'failed to respond to treatment', perhaps because the injury or the condition were too severe. Yet most surgical operations are not carried out as an emergency: they are carefully planned and performed to relieve symptoms or improve outlook in patients who spontaneously and willingly walk into hospital on their own two feet. If, a few days later, the patient is carried out of hospital in a wooden box after an operation has been performed, it is hard for the casual observer to avoid, consciously or subconsciously, linking such an outcome with the surgeon who did it.

If it is difficult for a third party to separate the outcome from the operation, and the operation from the operator, then it is doubly difficult, if not impossible, for the surgeons themselves to make such a separation in their own minds. I have worked as a surgeon surrounded by many other fellow surgeons for the past 25 years, and have never known a surgeon to take the loss of a patient lightly. That said, the reactions of surgeons to such events can be very interesting and very, very different, and this is often a reflection of their different personalities.

One of my finest trainees was an intelligent, softly spoken, and kind young Irishman called Andrew Drain. He tragically died of a virulent form of leukaemia before completing his specialist training. He had an unusually mature early interest in the psychology of the surgical mentality, and he and I once tried to categorise the reaction experienced by surgeons when they 'lose' a patient.

The closest we got to understanding these reactions was to recognise that the surgeons who experience them could be classified into one of two broad stereotypes. The first is a self-flagellator: this surgeon would go back over the case, reviewing every single detail, asking 'What if?' at every juncture, and self-blaming for any aspect of the patient management where care may have been anything but optimal. After an intense period of self-scrutiny, sadness, and bitterness, this surgeon draws a line under the events, and returns to work the following day, a little chastened and perhaps a little more careful. The second type would also go back over the case, reviewing every single detail, asking 'What if?' at every juncture, until the discovery and identification of a minor error or omission by somebody else. This type of surgeon is then absolutely convinced that the death is somebody else's fault, becomes visibly and palpably cheerful, and returns to work as if nothing had happened. I am not exaggerating: I still remember a senior surgeon who rushed into hospital on a Sunday night after his patient unexpectedly died. This was not in order to speak to bereaved relatives or provide moral support for his junior staff, but specifically to pore laboriously over the case notes of the recently deceased patient in the nurses' office. Twenty minutes later, he identified a minor electrolyte abnormality that was not, in his opinion, adequately dealt with by the hapless resident medical officer on call two nights previously. He looked up from the notes, turned to me, and said, 'Aha: *he* killed my patient', then smiled, got up, and went home to his gin and tonic, satisfied that his *amour-propre* was intact. This was not a cavalier surgeon, nor was he one who did not care for his patients. He was a hard-working, dedicated, and selfless man who devoted his life to surgery, but his behaviour here was driven by the need to restore self-confidence before facing the next operating day.

In a way, this is not all that surprising. Regardless of the coping mechanism employed, a surgeon must ensure that he or she is going to be able to function almost immediately after the tragedy. After all, other patients are awaiting treatment the very next day, and the day after that, and operations must be performed by competent and confident individuals who are capable of making correct decisions and making them quickly. The operating theatre is no room for indulging in excessive introspection and wallowing in the paralysis of all-pervasive self-doubt.

If all of the above is true, then it must apply with even greater poignancy when a death occurs not a day or two after surgery, but on the operating table itself. It is here that separating operator and operation from outcome is nigh impossible. And it is here that one would expect to find the most profound impact of the outcome of the last case on the outcome of the next one.

The issue first came to the fore in abdominal surgery, the branch of surgery that deals with the contents of the belly, such as the gall bladder and the intestines. Some abdominal surgery is carried out in desperate emergencies, such as when patients are brought in with the rupture of an internal organ and dangerous infections of the body cavity. These patients may arrive in the emergency room in a desperate state, with raging infection and failure of multiple organ systems, and it is not surprising if some of these patients die despite the best efforts of the surgeons. Most abdominal surgery, however, is routine, carefully planned, and carried out electively to remove a diseased gall bladder, fix a hernia, and so on. It is true that many patients who present for such surgery are elderly, and some may have heart and lung problems purely as a result of their age. Despite the worsening risk profile of these patients, advances in anaesthesia, monitoring, and the general overall care of the surgical patient have resulted in elective abdominal surgery becoming a very safe treatment indeed. All of this means that, in such elective surgery, the death of a patient on the operating table — an intra-operative death — is now a vanishingly rare event.

Rare events do sometimes happen, though, and they occasionally happen in rapid succession. In Scotland, one particular surgeon (and his hapless patients) had an almost incredible misfortune: having experienced the unexpected with the death of one patient on the operating table, he continued with the day's scheduled operating list only for another patient to suffer the same tragic fate. For two patients to die consecutively on an operating table was virtually unheard of, and, not surprisingly, the media took notice, and there was a clamorous outcry. One focus of the reaction to this bit of medical news was that many sections of the media found it incomprehensible that surgeons 'carried on regardless' with the day's work after such a calamity.

In the UK, a death during surgery must be reported to the appropriate authorities. The coroner's courts deals with such deaths in England, Wales, and Northern Ireland, while the procurators fiscal and sheriff courts deal with them in Scotland. These cases were duly reported to the local procurator fiscal, and were heard some time later in court. During the hearing in the Falkirk Sheriff Courthouse on 26 January 1999, some expert witnesses advised the court of their educated opinion that, after an intra-operative death, surgeons should cease operating that day. Sheriff Albert Sheehan listened to this advice, and recommended that the Scottish Royal Colleges and the Scottish Intercollegiate Guidelines Network should consider whether guidelines or advice were needed for surgeons to follow if they experience a death on the table. Should they carry on regardless? Should they take some time off?

At that stage, there was an utter lack of consensus on the matter. Opinions were divided, and appeared to be deeply held, but none of them was backed by the slightest shred of evidence. A survey of Welsh orthopaedic surgeons looked for some information about working after an intra-operative death. Among the survey participants, only one of 16 surgeons who had such a death actually cancelled further operations that day, but eight of the surgeons who experienced the death of a patient during surgery felt that some time without operating would have been advisable. Some cardiac surgeons (who, by the nature of their work, are more familiar with such events than their orthopaedic colleagues) said that they behaved differently after a death on the table, and many anaesthetists stated that if surgeons and their performance are affected by such an event, then their close colleagues, the anaesthetists, are equally affected, if not even more so. Questions were also asked about the rest of the operating team.

The events in Falkirk raised many questions that the medical profession had not previously addressed. Indeed, it was a question that we doctors did not know was there. Should we stop operating if a patient dies on the table?

There are many ways of addressing the issue, and many ancillary questions can be asked. A few of these are listed below:

- What actually happens in practice now? Do most surgeons stop or continue?
- In an ideal world, what should happen? Stop or carry on?
- Is there any proper, good reason based on evidence for surgeons to stop? In other words, will patients operated in the immediate aftermath of a death on the table fare worse than other patients?
- If the team stops, then for how long?
- Who should stop? Surgeons? Anaesthetists? Scrub nurses? The entire team? The whole hospital?

In cardiac surgery, a death on the operating table is still a rare event, but it certainly occurs far more often than in abdominal or orthopaedic surgery, or indeed in any other kind of surgical specialty. There are, of course, many reasons for this.

The most obvious reason is that the heart and the great vessels that pour into it or out of it are of course both big and full of blood. A tear or rupture, whether caused by disease, injury, or a surgeon's knife, can result in catastrophic bleeding. Your heart pumps your entire blood volume around your body once a minute, which means that a large hole in a heart chamber or a big blood vessel, while the heart is still beating, will result in 'bleeding out' in around one minute.

The second reason is to do with the heart itself. When an orthopaedic surgeon sets a broken bone, that bone, together with the limb within which it is situated, is rested in plaster until healing occurs. When a piece of bowel or stomach is taken out, the alimentary system is given a period of rest, with 'NIL BY MOUTH' instructions until the gut recovers. Almost every organ that is operated on is given a chance to rest and recover before it is expected to take up its duties once more. Not so the heart. The sick heart, made temporarily even sicker by being operated on, is simply expected to get on with it, and go back to work as soon as the operation is finished. This is mandatory: a patient whose heart does not work at all at the end of an operation is almost always a dead patient. (I say almost always, because we now have artificial hearts that can buy some time in the hope of a quick recovery of the real thing, but they are imperfect machines, risky to use, fraught with complications of their own, and ridiculously expensive.)

Sometimes, bleeding out and a non-functioning heart can happen together in the same patient. For such a patient, death is a double certainty.

Most heart surgeons will experience a death on the table at least once. One such heart surgeon, Stephen Large, is a colleague and friend of mine. He wrote an account of the death on the operating table of a young man, aged only 17, who died after a moderately high-risk operation (see Appendix B). In this account, he describes the events leading to the death, and the impact that these events have had on him many years later, which he calls a 'true haunting'. My own experience of death on the table is sharpest in relation to its immediate impact, and it is a feeling of catastrophic and absolute loneliness. When a patient dies on the table, everybody in the operating theatre is still physically present, but, to my mind, they have all simply disappeared. All that is left is the patient who has been failed, and the surgeon who has failed him or her, with the harsh glare of the operating-room light focused unforgivingly on us both.

As such a tragic event is a rare but regular feature of heart surgery, I felt that we heart surgeons were the ideally placed specialty to look into its impact and address the questions listed above. In particular, I wanted to find out if having a death on the table affects the performance of the surgeon immediately afterwards. I discussed the idea with Tony Goldstone and Chris Callaghan, who at the time were two promising surgical trainees in our department, and they were very keen on the concept. Together with Jon Mackay, an anaesthetist, and Susan Charman, a statistician, we designed a study to look into this question.

The first thing we set out to do was to ask cardiac surgeons and anaesthetists what their actual practices were. We sent questionnaires to all the senior cardiac surgeons and anaesthetists in the country. We first asked them if they had experienced a death on the table. We then asked them whether they had stopped work for a period afterwards. We also asked them, regardless of what they actually did after such a death, if they *thought* they should stop work for a period after such an event. We also asked them if they thought it would be helpful to be given some guidance as to what they should do after such an event. Finally, we gave them some free space to express their views on the subject.

The second thing we did was to seek some evidence to confirm or refute whether continuing to operate after a death on the table had an adverse effect on the outcomes of the patients who had their operations immediately afterwards (in the following 48 hours). We took all the patients who, within 48 hours after a death on the table, were operated by the same surgeon who had experienced that death, and tried to see how their outcomes compared with patients operated at other, more 'normal' times.

The results of both the survey of surgeons and anaesthetists and of the outcome comparison were published in the *British Medical Journal* (Goldstone 2004). Some of our findings were predictable, but others were a complete surprise.

The survey was a very successful one, in that of just under 500 senior surgeons and anaesthetists who were approached, 76 per cent responded. This is an exceptionally large proportion for an anonymous and optional postal survey, and indicates that the subject was one about which people felt strongly enough to want their opinion heard.

The majority of surgeons (86 per cent) and anaesthetists (95 per cent) had encountered at least one death on the table. Just over half of the surgeons (53 per cent), but only around one in five (22 per cent) of the anaesthetists, actually stopped work immediately afterwards. Both surgeons and anaesthetists cited fatigue, emotion, medico-legal concerns, and the advice of colleagues as reasons to stop. Most of these doctors felt that guidelines would be helpful to them.

We had given the survey participants the opportunity for freehand comment so that they could express their own thoughts on the subject, and one salient topic came up repeatedly. Most of those who said that they wanted guidelines also commented that, in their view, it is important that such guidelines make a crucial distinction between the types of death on the table. To paraphrase the feelings expressed by the majority: if the death on the table was to some extent 'expected', in other words a high-risk or emergency death, then it doesn't matter too much, but, if the death on the table was totally unexpected, such as in low-risk elective surgery, then stopping and taking stock is probably a good idea.

This is what the professionals thought. Now for the evidence: the study aimed to find if those patients operated in the immediate aftermath of a death on the table fared differently from other patients. We identified a total of 81 deaths on the table at Papworth Hospital during the five-year study period. At first glance, that may sound like a lot, but bear in mind that Papworth performs about 2,000 operations per year, so that would be a lot less than 1 per cent chance of dying on the table during the period of the study.

In the 48 hours immediately after a death on the table, 233 patients were operated by the very same surgeons who had just experienced the death. These were the patients we were interested in: were their outcomes affected? When we compared them to virtually identical patients in every respect who were *not* operated immediately after a death, we found that there was no difference in survival rates. We did, however, find that these 233 patients had more complications and spent longer in hospital than their peers. Clearly, therefore, a death on the table does affect performance, but not enough to endanger the life of the next patient.

So far, all of the above, if not exactly predictable, can be described as not all that surprising. The real surprise comes next.

Our survey of the profession had indicated that a death that was to some extent 'expected' (high risk or emergency) should not matter so much, but that a death that was a bolt from the blue (low risk, elective) should be followed with caution and introspection. With the survey finding in mind, we subdivided the 233 patients operated immediately after a death into two groups: those preceded by a high-risk or emergency death (in other words, a somewhat 'expected' death) and those preceded by a low-risk or elective death (in other words, an unexpected, bolt-from-the-blue death). Here the result was astounding: patients operated on after a death that was somewhat to be 'expected' fared worse, and had a higher mortality than those operated on after an unexpected, low-risk death. This was exactly the opposite of what the professionals thought.

We do not know why this is so, though I suspect that once again it has something to do with the personality of surgeons, which I explore in the next chapter. What we do know, however, is that a death on the table does indeed have an impact on subsequent performance. At the very least, there are longer hospital stays due to complications, even if overall mortality is not affected. And those hoped-for guidelines? We are, of course, still waiting for them.

up, ready for the next heartbeat. When the ventricle begins to beat in order to pump the blood to the body, the valve shuts tight to prevent back-flow, so that all the blood is pumped forward into the aorta to supply the body with oxygen and goodness.

The mitral valve is vulnerable in rheumatic fever, a medical condition that tends to happen in childhood, and begins with a simple sore throat caused by a fairly common bug from a family of bacteria called streptococcus. The body's immune system reacts to this streptococcus infection by mounting a vigorous defence, sending white cells and antibodies to destroy the alien invader. Unfortunately, the powerful immune response to this particular streptococcus is not very selective, and sometimes attacks the body's own tissues, especially the joints (hence the 'rheumatic' part of the fever), but also, incomprehensibly, the heart valves, including the mitral valve. As a result of this attack, the valve becomes horribly inflamed and, later, scarred as the body tries to repair the damage. As the years pass, this scarring progressively becomes thicker and harder. The leaflets of the valve, normally gossamer-thin and flexible, become thick, unwieldy, and calcified. Finally, the leaflets end up fused into an ugly, craggy white rock with a tiny slit in the middle. Through this slit, five litres of blood are somehow supposed to pass every minute if the patient is to stay alive, and, not surprisingly, this is an untenable situation. Gradually, pressure rises upstream of this narrowed valve. This high pressure in the left atrium backs up into the lungs and into the right side of the heart, the veins of the body, and the liver, all of which are upstream of the valve. The lungs begin to leak and the right heart fails, the liver and legs swell up, and the patient becomes tired, very breathless, and in a poor shape indeed. The only way to relieve the symptoms is by having the mitral valve open properly again, but, as it is deep within the heart, fixing it without a heart–lung machine is virtually impossible.

Virtually impossible is not, however, impossible. Pioneering heart surgeons actually found a way before the invention of the heart–lung machine, and that operation is closed mitral valvotomy. Here is the recipe, but please do not try this at home:

- Put the patient to sleep.
- Open the left chest.
- Place a circular or 'purse-string' stitch around a finger-sized area of the left atrium.
- Make a cut within this purse-string.
- Push a finger quickly into the cut before the patient bleeds out, and tighten the purse-string around the finger.
- Wiggle finger around the atrium, feeling for the mitral valve, and the tight slit within it.
- Once found, shove finger into the slit and tear it, to widen the opening (do this quickly: while your finger is blocking the slit, there is no circulation). If necessary, you can use a dilator to open the valve further.
- Pull your finger out, and quickly pull the purse-string tight and tie it shut.
- Heave a sigh of relief: job done.
- Close the chest and open a can of applause.

Henry Souttar was the first surgeon to carry this out successfully in London, as far back as 1925, but it was probably an American in Philadelphia, Charles Bailey, who convinced the world that there was some merit in this apparently crazy, desperate procedure. Bailey first tried out mitral valvotomy on four patients, and killed every single one of them. As a result, he was banned from operating in three hospitals in the Philadelphia area. Undaunted, in 1948, he decided to have another go. He planned to operate on two more patients on the same day, but in two different hospitals. His rationale for this strategy was most disturbing. He figured out that if the first patient died at one hospital, he could rush across town and get the second operation started at the other hospital before the news broke out and he was banned from operating at these hospitals as well. The morning patient died on the operating table, but the afternoon patient survived, and the operation became established. As you have probably surmised, this is hairy surgery. It requires supreme confidence, nerves of steel, and fast decision-making, but, compared to the next operation I shall tell you about, closed mitral valvotomy is a walk in the park.

The condition of atrial septal defect, or ASD, is a relatively common congenital abnormality. In this, the baby is born with a hole between the right atrium and the left atrium, which are just upstream of the right and left ventricles. The two atria should not communicate at all, as they are naturally separated by a wall, which is called the atrial septum. There is a good reason for this separation, and it is easy to understand. This is how blood circulates through the heart:

Having been around the body to deliver oxygen and food, the blue and useless oxygen-poor blood comes back to the heart and lungs to be loaded with oxygen and pumped around the body again. This is its journey:

- collect in the right atrium
- move to the right ventricle
- get pumped to the lungs to pick up oxygen
- collect in the left atrium (now the blood is pink and carries oxygen)

- move to the left ventricle
- get pumped to the body
- deliver the oxygen to the body (now the blood is blue and without oxygen)
- come back to the right atrium and start the cycle all over again.

So, to simplify the journey, it goes like this:

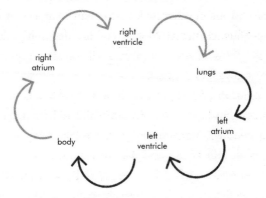

When a hole exists in the wall or septum between the atria, the blood flow changes to this:

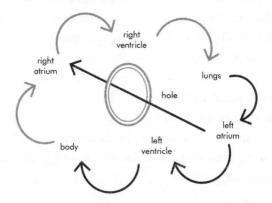

As you can see, a lot of the blood ends up going round in circles: right atrium, right ventricle, lungs, right atrium, right ventricle, lungs, and so on. This is a terrible waste of the heart's pumping energy. The right ventricle ends up having to pump twice or three times as much blood just to keep the flow going around the body at an acceptable level. Not being designed to do this, the right ventricle fails. As for the lungs, they end up handling twice or three times as much blood going through them as necessary, their blood pressure rises, and they eventually fail.

Babies who are born with an ASD appear perfectly normal to begin with, and usually have a normal early childhood, but their right ventricles and lungs are overworking every minute of the day and night. Gradually, the right ventricle and the lungs begin to fail, and, sometime in childhood, adolescence, or young adulthood, patients with ASD become short of breath, and that is when they come to the attention of doctors. The doctors examine the patients, do a few tests, and the hole is found.

Closing an ASD is no great surgical challenge. It's only a hole, after all, and it takes a competent surgeon no more than about five to 20 minutes with a stitch to cobble it up or patch it, but, in order to reach it, you have to open the right atrium. Do this without a heart–lung machine and without isolating the heart from the circulation, and the patient's lifeblood ends up on the floor.

Before the heart–lung machine was invented, the pioneering heart surgeons of the 1930s and 1940s tried a variety of methods to get at the hole 'blind', without actually opening the atrium to see it. They finger-pushed the wall of the atrium into the hole and tried to cobble it from outside 'by feel'. They tried to insert plugs and other devices to block the hole. They developed many ingenious methods, some of which worked partially, and some of which did not work at all, but all of them had an appalling mortality rate. Then someone had the great idea of clamping the two huge veins that pour into the right atrium, opening it, and closing the hole very, very quickly. The reason for this need for speed is that, during that time, there is no circulation, and the brain and the patient are both rapidly dying. As we know, the brain will only survive the absence of circulation for a few minutes. To help prolong the period of zero-circulation that the patient will tolerate without brain damage, it seemed a good idea to cool the body and the brain before the circulation is stopped.

Finally, on 2 September 1952, in Minnesota, USA, surgeon John Lewis made this operation a reality. Together with three assistants (Richard Varco, Mansur Taufic, and Walton Lillehei), Lewis operated on a five-year-old girl with an ASD. They put the little girl to sleep and cooled her from normal body temperature of 37°C to 28°C with refrigerated blankets. They then opened the chest, and clamped the great veins that flow into the right atrium. They opened the right atrium, sucked out the blood that was in it, quickly stitched up the hole, hastily closed the right atrium, and took off the clamps. The heart started pumping again. They re-warmed the girl, and she survived, without brain damage, after a period of zero circulation that lasted only five and a half minutes. The girl was cured of her ASD, and her operation was the world's first successful procedure on the open human heart under direct vision. This marked the beginning of the era of open-heart surgery. A couple of years later, the heart–lung machine was invented, and heart surgery took off.

When John Lewis died in 1993, his fellow surgeon during that seminal operation Walton Lillehei said 'From that memorable beginning in Minneapolis, open-heart surgery has grown to be one of the major medical contributions of the 20th century. In the past year, worldwide, more than one open-heart operation was done every minute! Such was the legacy that John left.'

Interestingly, Lillehei went on to pioneer many innovations in heart surgery, the most notable of which was the use of a human being as a heart–lung machine! He operated on many children by using one of their parents as a machine to keep the child's circulation going. Both parent and child were anaesthetised, and tubes attached to connect the child to the mother or father's circulation, as though the child was an extra 'organ' of the parent. Under these circumstances, the child's heart could be isolated from the circulation and fixed, while the parent's heart, lungs, and circulation kept the child alive. This type of operation must be one of the very few that can actually have a 200 per cent mortality rate, in that it can kill the patient and the mother or father of the patient (and occasionally, it did).

I have segued into the early milestones of heart surgery for a good reason, and that is to illustrate clearly that the very nature of the specialty in those days attracted a very particular type of surgeon: an adventurer, a risk-taker, a daredevil, a pioneering, determined, ruthless, and courageous sort of person with no room for lengthy introspection or nagging self-doubt. These were almost universally the attributes of the pioneering cardiac surgeon's personality, and some of these traits still remain in evidence in some heart surgeons to this day.

So what do we know about this side of surgeons' personality characteristics? And more specifically, does it have an impact on their results, which are, after all, what we care about?

Psychologists are fond of describing and classifying people according to various psychological and personality traits. In a way, the father of medicine, Hippocrates, was something of a personality psychologist. He believed that the body fluids, or 'humours', were responsible for our psychological make-up. Blood makes us animated and confident (sanguine), phlegm causes us to be cool and detached (phlegmatic), yellow bile makes us bitter and twisted (jaundiced), and black bile causes us to be depressed and miserable (melancholic). Modern-day psychology recognises these and many other personality types and personality traits. Some of these are well known to the layperson, such as extrovert versus introvert, analytical versus intuitive, and so on. Of course, many different aspects of personality can be studied and assessed. More recently, there has been a heightened interest in the particular trait of personality that determines how willing an individual is to take risk. This is known as 'risk propensity', and much of the interest in it has arisen as a result of the impact it can have on decisions made in the financial and managerial worlds, where it is self-evident that excessive risk takers, such as rogue traders or bankers, may lead their organisations into financial ruin.

But risk propensity plays a major part in surgery and its outcomes, too — not least in heart surgery. We have seen in this chapter that pioneering heart surgeons were gung-ho risk-taking daredevils. They had to be: without taking at least some risk, no progress would have been possible. One who is petrified by fire will never blaze a trail.*

I suspected that this risk-taking culture could be seen in the personality traits and behaviour of some surgeons more than others. If it could be seen, it could be measured. So I decided to ask the heart surgeons at Papworth Hospital to locate themselves

---

* We should pause briefly to pay tribute to those patients who willingly submitted themselves to these trailblazing procedures. Whereas surgeons undoubtedly took risks with their careers, futures, and standing within the medical community, their patients took the ultimate and far greater risk: they gambled with their lives. They fully deserve our admiration and respect.

and their fellow surgeons on a scale representing the range of risk propensity. I did this by distributing a survey that asked participants to use a visual analogue scale that ranged from one extreme (no risk-taking whatsoever, whatever the situation) to another (taking crazy risks all the time).

Here is the visual analogue scale as presented in the survey:

Name of Surgeon: ....

X

1   2   3   4   5   6   7   8   9   10

←-------------------   ------------------→

Excessively Risk Averse   Excessively Risk-taking
Triple-checks Everything   'Cowboy'
Anally Retentive   Flies by the Seat of Pants
Obsessive-compulsive   Cuts Corners

Participants were asked to answer the question for every surgeon at Papworth by placing an 'X' to indicate where each surgeon fell, in their opinion, on the risk-propensity scale. Both extremes of the scale were made to look equally unpleasant and negative, so that surgeons would not be placed towards the ends unless they were truly perceived to be deviant. All the surgeons themselves, as well as a group of anaesthetists and assistants who worked very closely with them, filled in the survey, so that, in total, I had 29 responses about the 13 senior surgeons who work at my hospital. This is what the survey showed:

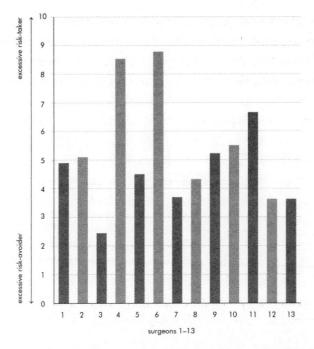

As you can see, there are marked differences. We have two or perhaps three surgeons who can most assuredly be described as risk-taking cowboys, and one who is firmly ensconced in a mouse hole at the obsessive-compulsive opposite end of the scale. In a way, this is not at all surprising. Like all human beings, surgeons differ in many aspects of their personality traits, and risk propensity is simply yet another personality trait. The question that immediately springs to mind is which of these, if any, is associated with better clinical outcomes. The quickest way of doing this is to look at risk-adjusted mortality ratios, or RAMR. This is simply the ratio between actual mortality and expected mortality, expressed as a decimal number. If the ratio is 1.0, the outcome is exactly as expected. If it is less than 1.0, actual mortality is lower than expected.

At the time of the survey, the average RAMR for all surgeons taken together was 0.22. The most extreme risk avoider in my survey is surgeon 3, whose RAMR is 0.1, a very good result. Next come surgeons 12 and 13: their RAMRs are 0.4 and zero, respectively. Looking at the most risk-taking surgeons, they are surgeons 4, 6, and 11. Their RAMRs are 0.25, 0.6, and 0.25. The surgeons in the middle of the scale also have wide variation in their RAMRs, ranging from zero to 0.33. There seems to be no correlation whatsoever between risk propensity and successful outcomes. We have risk-takers and risk-avoiders achieving broadly similar results, with similar variations within each group. So there is no association between individual surgeons' risk propensity and the outcomes for their patients. The average results at Papworth are excellent overall. Some of our surgeons perform slightly better or slightly worse than our average, but this appears to be totally unrelated to their individual risk propensity: a personality trait that shows a propensity to take risk or a propensity to avoid it does not appear to directly influence outcomes.

One might be a little disappointed by this seemingly negative finding. After all, there is good evidence that it is obsessive risk avoidance that has made aviation so safe, and that one of the problems in medicine is the comparative dearth of such risk avoidance. One would naturally expect that excessively risk-taking surgeons should encounter more problems, and therefore have worse results. The facts suggest otherwise. Does that mean that risk propensity has no bearing at all on surgical outcomes?

It would be perfectly reasonable to postulate that a surgeon's propensity to take risk is not immutably etched in concrete. Regardless of his or her position on the risk propensity scale, our surgeon is likely to vary in risk-taking within a certain range. I, for one, know that I am sometimes more gung-ho than at other times.

Sometimes, I am adventurous. At other times, I am hyper-careful. The variation in my own risk propensity seems to be directly related to the life events I am experiencing at the time.

Does this variation in risk propensity apply to everyone? Common sense would suggest that it probably does. A driver who has just been caught for speeding is more likely to observe the speed limit. A smoker whose best friend has just died of lung cancer is more likely to consider ditching the cigarettes. An investor who has just lost a tidy sum on the stock market is unlikely to feel bullish when the next risky investment opportunity presents itself. We are human, and our behaviour is strongly modified by our reaction to certain events. I am not making this up: cognitive psychologists have studied these phenomena for years, and there is even a branch of science called 'heuristics', which focuses on the link between experience, learning, and behaviour. Furthermore, evolutionary psychologists believe that this type of judgement bias is actually hardwired in our genes, and can be explained in Darwinian evolutionary terms. There are some truly peculiar traits in our behaviour towards risky situations. Some of these traits do not even make sense, but we guess that they are there because they must have been in some way beneficial for survival in the ancestral environment 100,000 years ago or thereabouts. As a result, certain types of events in your life make you more risk-averse than usual, and happenings of another kind make you more gung-ho than usual.

Let us now come back to surgeons. We know that, like every other group of professionals, surgeons come in all shapes and sizes: male and female, short and tall, fat and thin, black and white. We have also established that they differ in personality, and, in particular, we now know for certain that they differ in their position on the risk propensity scale. I also know that there is not a shred of evidence that sex, size, and colour have any impact at all on surgeon performance, though it seems reasonable that a surgeon's age, experience, manual dexterity, conscientiousness, knowledge, and sound judgement may influence surgical outcomes. These factors are likely to have an impact, but what about the small variation in an individual surgeon's risk propensity? Does that affect the results of surgery?

Recall those two studies that had somewhat surprising findings. In the study of deaths on the operating table, we found that such a death did in fact have an adverse impact on surgical performance in the subsequent 48 hours, so that patients operated on in the immediate aftermath of an on-table death fared worse than others. This in itself was predictable, but what was surprising was that the effect appeared to be worse if the preceding death on the table was a high-risk or emergency (somewhat 'expected') death. In fact, this finding was diametrically opposite to the views of the clinicians who were surveyed about the subject, and who overwhelmingly believed with conviction that an unexpected death in a low-risk patient is precisely the sort of thing that can affect subsequent performance.

The second study looked at holidays and surgical performance. Here there were no expectations. One could envisage that a break would do the surgeon some good, and deliver him or her refreshed and raring to go, but one could equally well imagine that a long time away from the operating table would deliver an uncertain surgeon who has been somewhat de-skilled and who will perform a little worse until back in the groove. The findings showed that there was no loss of skill after a holiday, and that results were, if anything, better than usual on the first day back. This in itself was not too surprising, but the outcomes of patients operated the day *before* a surgeon went on holiday were surprisingly bad: the mortality of these patients was more than double the mortality of those operated on the first day back from holiday.

We do not know the true cause behind these unexpected findings, but here is a possible explanation for both.

We have established that surgeons vary in their risk propensity. We know that this variation between surgeons does not by itself relate to variation in outcomes. We also know that the risk propensity of an individual surgeon is not fixed, but varies in a way that is affected by the events of life, so that each surgeon's risk propensity spans a range. So perhaps surgeons are safest and best when they are operating towards the risk-averse end of their own personal risk-propensity range.

Consider a hypothetical surgeon in action within the context of the two previous studies. He is an ordinary bloke, with a risk-propensity range somewhere in the middle. He is neither an excessive risk-taker nor so obsessively risk-averse that he is paralysed with fear in the operating room. Most days, he works in the middle of his risk-propensity range, then something happens that moves him to one or the other end of his range. Let us look at some scenarios.

Scenario 1

Our surgeon is on call for emergencies, and is presented with an almost impossibly high-risk patient. The situation is one of kill-or-cure salvage: he either operates immediately or the patient will die. It is 10.00 p.m. Many people feel the case is hopeless. In fact, he knows of many colleagues who would not dream of offering surgery to a patient of such high risk, but he also knows that, without his intervention, the patient will be dead soon. He decides to go ahead. There are both expected difficulties and unexpected complications. The operation takes 12 hours instead of four hours, as would normally be the case. He is up all night. His routine, next day's operating list of two straightforward CABG operations is going to be delayed. At 10.00 a.m. the following day, he has tried everything to save the emergency patient, and all his efforts have failed. He has been 'firefighting' all night, and finally decides to give up, as the situation is hopeless. The patient dies on the operating table. He sends for the next routine CABG case, and is ready to start operating at about 11.00 a.m. He is very tired, and slightly fed up with the way the night has turned out, but wants to get on and finish these 'easy' cases as quickly as possible so he can get home and rest before the dinner party he has promised to attend. As he now embarks on the routine case, with a 'bring 'em on' attitude, is he likely to be more risk averse or risk-taking? I believe he is undoubtedly going to be taking more risks than usual.

Scenario 2

Our same surgeon has been having a good run, with great results. He is happily operating on a low-risk young patient in a relaxed and pleasant environment. The operation is easy, and he is enjoying operating-room banter with the staff when something suddenly and unexpectedly goes catastrophically wrong. The otherwise fit and healthy patient, who had rightfully expected a normal life span after correction of a heart defect, dies on the operating table: an unmitigated and totally unexpected disaster. The next case is a standard CABG operation. When he approaches it, is he likely to be more risk averse or risk-taking? Of course he is going to be risk-averse. In fact, he will be terrified: he has had the rug pulled out from under him, and has been left questioning and doubting everything, including himself and his purpose in life. He will certainly not be taking risks.

Scenario 3

Our surgeon is operating on the last day before a much-needed two-week holiday in the sun. He and his family have a flight to catch at 7.00 p.m. that very evening, but he thinks he will finish operating in time to get home and help with the packing. There are other important last-minute arrangements to be made, such as to book parking at the airport and fill the car with fuel. Sadly, that is not all: there is a large pile of patient correspondence to be dealt with before he goes, and he knows that, if it is not dealt with now, it will have grown to unmanageable proportions on his return. Added to all of that are a couple of administrative meetings that simply must be squeezed in over lunch before his leave begins. He has not had a break from work for three months, and this holiday is so important to him. His mind is already on the flight and the beach, but these cases must be operated first. Is he likely to be taking risks? Definitely.

Scenario 4

Our surgeon has just spent two weeks on a fantastic holiday in the sun. Surgery, administrative work, and hospital-management problems seem miles away. He is re-acquainted with his loved ones, with himself, and with what he really enjoys doing when he is not operating. He is back, refreshed, and happy but has not set foot in an operating room for more than two weeks. It's Monday morning, the first patient is on the table, and our surgeon hopes that he is still up to the task (especially since he found out on his return that the patient he operated on the day before his leave did not do so well). Does he take risks? Obviously not: he will be at his most risk-averse.

In scenario 2, a young patient died unexpectedly on the operating table, and, in scenario 4, the surgeon is a tad uncertain about his ability to operate after a long absence. Both contribute to a mindset that is hyper-aware of what can go wrong, and both engender extra care to avoid errors. This is analogous to the situation with Jehovah's Witnesses. By categorically refusing blood transfusion, they take away from the surgeon the possibility of giving blood in case of bleeding, and thus withdraw one of the surgeon's safety nets. A surgeon faced with a Jehovah's Witness on the operating table is naturally going to be more risk-averse when it comes to bleeding, and will take a lot of care to ensure that the risk of bleeding is minimised. It is no surprise that such patients bleed so little.

If my hunch is true, and surgeons are safest and best when they are operating towards the risk-averse end of their own personal risk-propensity range, it goes a long way to explain both the surprising findings in the holiday study and the study of deaths on the table. It also means that we have at our disposal a new method to improve surgical outcomes, over and above good training, good technique, conscientiousness, and a high standard of care, over and above robust quality monitoring and even the Hawthorne effect: we should be able to improve surgical outcomes by modifying the risk-taking behaviour of surgeons. How do we do this? I am not exactly sure yet, but I have a few ideas. For a start, we need a hard measure of risk propensity, one that is more robust than surgeons' own perception of themselves and others, and we also need a host of interventions specifically designed to modify such propensity. Preliminary exploratory work suggests that all of this may indeed be possible, but it is beyond the scope of this book, and will form the basis of some future research on this fascinating topic. In other words, watch this space.

10

The Future of Medicine

Healthcare is serious business. Sometimes, it is deadly serious. It is also big business. Regardless of the way that healthcare is provided and financed (private or public, via taxes, insurance, or dirty cash), most civilised countries spend somewhere in the region of 10 per cent of their gross domestic product (GDP) on the health of their citizens. This is an astounding proportion of national spending. It means that one dollar (or pound or euro) of every ten that the nation earns goes on healthcare.

In the case of Britain, the NHS budget is currently around £130 billion per year, or £247,337 every minute. Despite this apparent profligacy, Britain is considered to be a relative skinflint in this area of public expenditure, in that it spends only a miserly 9 per cent of its GDP on health.* France is on around 12 per cent, and the USA is on a whopping 18 per cent of GDP. The trend for all of these percentages goes inexorably upwards as nations become richer, and their citizens live longer and expect more and better healthcare.

---

* Though it is not alone: Portugal, Finland, and Australia, for instance, have similar figures.

These massive figures and their huge impact on the budgets of nations and the pockets of taxpayers inevitably mean that healthcare must be managed in some way to ensure that the prodigious sums of money spent on it at least yield a reasonable outcome for the patients. This is purely from a financial point of view. Of course, the case for decent and intelligent management of healthcare goes beyond the mere financial: the outcomes affect people, their health, lives, and happiness, and, by implication, the lives and happiness of those around them.

So the managers and the management consultants entered the fray. To begin with, they were driven primarily or perhaps solely by a desire to reduce the costs of healthcare, and they predictably started by looking at the bottom line.

During the early years of the Thatcher government, spending on healthcare in the UK barely exceeded 3 per cent of GDP. This meant that Britain was spending far, far less than comparable developed countries. Waiting lists were interminably long, many patients did not receive basic treatment, and those who did had to wait a very long time for such treatment, sometimes as much as one or two years. We are not talking about the luxury end of medical treatment here, but about the bread and butter of therapies that the citizens of wealthy economies have come to expect: heart surgery, hip replacement, prostate operations, and so on. The conservative government under Thatcher decided that it would be a good idea to overhaul the health service, and make it more efficient, so as to obtain the best possible outcomes for the nation's tax contributions: value for money. What that government had not (or pretended it had not) realised was that it already owned, by and large, an excellent and highly efficient national health service, whose primary problem was starvation of resources, and what it had set out to do in overhauling the management of the service was akin to the driver of a fantastic supercar who, on having difficulties in starting the engine one morning, proceeds to dismantle and rebuild the engine without glancing at the fuel gauge reading 'EMPTY'.

So the government decided to change the entire structure of the health service, and to find ways of reducing costs by having expensive hospitals learn from cheaper ones. To this end, the government hired the services of a firm of very expensive and successful accountants and management consultants to improve the efficiency of the service, and these clever folk thought the best place to start would be cardiac surgery, because the specialty did relatively few types of operations in relatively large numbers, counted these operations, and had a reasonable idea of their costs and success rates. One of their first investigations was to compare the costs of cardiac surgery in two hospitals located in the same region of England. We shall call them hospital A and hospital B. The accountants calculated the costs of standard heart operations in these two hospitals for three broad types of operation: the first was CABG, the second included straightforward heart valve operations, and the third consisted of more difficult stuff: complex and combined operations, and 'redo' procedures (done on patients who have already had heart operations previously, which makes everything more hazardous). This is what they found:

	Hospital A	Hospital B
CABG	£5,600	£6,800
valve	£6,400	£8,700
redo/complex	£9,950	£4,800

The accountants looked at these figures, and drew what conclusions they could from them. They saw that hospital A was more cost-effective in simple CABG and valve operations, but that hospital B was more cost-effective in complicated and redo operations. They recommended that hospital A should stick to the basics, and that hospital B should be developed into a specialist tertiary-referral centre for the really complicated stuff, as it was so cost-effective in such cases.

Of course, these clever accountants never looked beyond the bottom line. Had they bothered to check the clinical outcomes in these two hospitals, they would have found a different story. Here are the mortality rates for the same operations in the two hospitals:

	Hospital A	Hospital B
CABG	3%	5%
valve	6%	11%
redo/complex	9%	65%*

* of whom 40 per cent died on the table

Therefore, the reason hospital B was so 'cost-effective' in treating complex patients is a simple one: many died on the operating table. In a high-risk patient, this is a very inexpensive pathway: it results in a very short hospital stay, no intensive care bills, and no recovery costs. The lesson from this appalling exercise is simple, and it is one emphasised earlier in this book. If we are interested in measuring and managing healthcare, we must measure those things that matter. Survival is an outcome of healthcare that should at least be as important as cost. In fact, there is very little point in measuring the cost of any intervention or other form of therapy until we know for sure that the therapy is effective. Once we know that, we can assess its cost-effectiveness and compare it to other forms of treatment.

It is now more than a quarter of a century since the escapades of those particular accountants, and we have learned much about the measurement of the quality of care. We still, sometimes, make the same old mistake of according too much importance to what is measurable. There is also room for improvement in our efforts to find robust ways of measuring that which is important. Despite these advances, we in healthcare continue to sin against the above rule, and one of the biggest errors committed by the bodies that seek to regulate medical care is a very elementary one: an obsession with process over outcome.

Let me explain. What is important in healthcare for the patient (the person who matters) is the *outcome* of treatment, and not the *process* by which the treatment is given. Unfortunately, outcomes can sometimes be difficult to measure. They are affected by risk profile and are subject to statistical vagaries. Process, however, is very easy to measure (especially if you choose those bits of it which are easily measurable). This means that scores of bodies regulating healthcare can introduce myriad rules about the way things are done, from the method of greeting a patient on arrival, the way a consent form is filled in, the colour of uniforms of healthcare staff, whether all doctors and nurses wear badges, whether dozens of tedious forms are filled in correctly, all the way to the colour of the cups and saucers used in the out-patient department. In the UK, the Department of Health has even dictated the type of font used in hospital signs to direct patients and visitors to various departments, and even mandated the colour and shape of headers used in the paper correspondence between doctors. Unfortunately, it does not stop there.

Under the Labour government at the turn of the millennium, the Department of Health in the UK decided that CABG should be a priority treatment, and introduced a target for managers: no patient on the waiting list for CABG should wait more than 13 weeks. Many in the developed world would choke on their coffee if they read about such an apparently unambitious target, and would be surprised that any wait whatsoever is considered acceptable for treatment that can be lifesaving in some patients, but you have to remember that, under the previous Conservative government, waiting times for CABG were often longer than 13 months.

So far, so good: reducing waiting times for CABG is a good thing — or so it would seem at first, but let us consider the different types of CABG. At one end of the spectrum, a patient can have a single coronary artery that has been completely blocked. This patient has angina, and wants a CABG to relieve the pain and restore a normal quality of life. As the artery has been completely blocked, it cannot get worse, and that patient is safe no matter how long the wait is. At the other end of the spectrum, another patient has 99 per cent narrowings in all his coronary arteries, including what is called the left main stem, which is the very beginning of the all-important left coronary artery, before a single branch has taken off. If the left main stem is blocked, two-thirds of the heart muscle dies, and so does the patient. In more than 20 years of practice, I have only ever seen two patients survive a blockage of the left main stem: after such a blockage, there is simply not enough heart muscle left to sustain the circulation. A tight narrowing in the left main stem is the sword of Damocles. This patient is also treated with a CABG. The Department of Health target does not distinguish between the two.

Let us now look at another condition: tight narrowing of the aortic valve. Wear and tear, among other things, causes the aortic valve on the exit from the heart to become narrowed. The heart copes by working extra hard to push the blood through, and the patient feels fine for years. Sooner or later, the heart runs out of energy reserves, and begins to fail. The patient then becomes short of breath, and develops other symptoms. When that happens, it means that the heart is at the end of its tether, and heart failure and death are just around the corner. This is another sword of Damocles.

A patient who has both a tight narrowing in the left main stem coronary artery and a tight narrowing in the aortic valve has two swords of Damocles above his head, and the strings that hold them are seriously frayed. This patient needs both an aortic valve replacement and a CABG, and he really needs them quickly, before one of the swords plunges into him. Under the Department of Health's 13-week CABG target, this patient is pushed to the back of the queue to make way for the CABG patient with a single blocked artery, for a very simple reason: a combined aortic valve operation plus CABG is not considered a CABG. Has this happened in real life? Yes, it has. Have patients died as a result? Yes, they have.

The above is a simple example of a target, based on what is measurable and introduced in good faith, resulting in worse outcomes for patients. Once again, obsession with process has trumped care about outcomes.

This type of distortion, which negates what matters by paying attention to what does not matter, pales into utter insignificance when one looks at what happened at a hospital in Staffordshire. The 'Mid Staffordshire NHS Foundation Trust' is a stupid managerial name for a hospital in the town of Stafford in England. This hospital failed abysmally in its duty of care to patients. Standards were so poor that it is estimated that several hundred patients (as many as 1,200 by some estimates) died needlessly under the 'care' of this hospital. The scandal was so large that a major parliamentary inquiry was launched, led by Sir Robert Francis. The final report of the Francis inquiry was published in

February 2013, and ran to 1,781 pages. It identified many failings, poor standards, and almost wilful, downright cruelty to patients. One of the most prominent among these failings was the slavish adherence to ill-conceived targets. Sir Robert Francis wrote (my italic emphasis):

> This was primarily caused by a serious failure on the part of a provider Trust Board. It did not listen sufficiently to its patients and staff or ensure the correction of deficiencies brought to the Trust's attention. Above all, it failed to tackle an insidious negative culture involving a tolerance of poor standards and a disengagement from managerial and leadership responsibilities. *This failure was in part the consequence of allowing a focus on reaching national access targets, achieving financial balance and seeking foundation trust status to be at the cost of delivering acceptable standards of care.*

Mid Staffordshire was an extreme example where obsession with process has undermined care about outcomes, but we unfortunately still see such distortions to a greater or lesser degree throughout healthcare. These distortions and their consequences illustrate the hidden and unexpected dangers of allowing managers and politicians to choose what is important about healthcare. If we clinicians want to protect our patients and hospitals from the deleterious effects of such distortions, we have to determine ourselves what we are trying to achieve, find a way of measuring whether or not we achieve it, and make that the criterion by which our performance is measured. In other words: make what's important measurable!

Despite these horror stories, at least in my specialty of cardiac surgery, we have made some important early progress. We are now good at measuring an outcome that really matters: survival. We can compare it with predicted survival, adjusting all measurements for each patient's risk profile, and we can come up with sensible, statistically sound comparisons to guide us towards identifying problems, fixing them, and running a rudimentary quality-control programme. It is true that we still tend to focus largely on the important but somewhat crude outcomes of death and survival, but at least we do recognise that other clinical outcomes also matter. Now that the immediate mortality rate from heart surgery is vanishingly small for most patients, perhaps it is time we started to use other measures of successful outcome, such as the patient being free from symptoms and the need for future interventions, having a good quality of life, and surviving not just the operation, but in the long term. We may, also, now begin to look seriously at the cost of treatment, so that we can deliver true healthcare improvements at the lowest possible price.

Medical practice as a whole also now needs to embrace the concepts that I outline in this book. The bulk of our discussion so far has concentrated on heart surgery. This is for several reasons. First, I am heart surgeon, and therefore know a little more about the topic than other medical specialties. Second, heart surgery has blazed the trail in quality monitoring, and, where it has led, others are following or will follow. Third, measuring outcomes in heart surgery is relatively straightforward, because there is one outcome that is simple, objective, directly related to the operation, and difficult to quibble about: death (or survival, if you prefer). So, if heart surgery patients come in alive, then they leave the hospital either alive or dead. There is no halfway house, and counting the live ones on exit is very easy indeed.

The trouble with specialists in other fields of medicine is that they (or so they claim) have no such clearly defined outcome measure. How on Earth would you measure the outcomes of treatments given by a psychiatrist, or a chest physician, or a kidney specialist, or even a bone surgeon operating on dodgy hip joints? Impossible, say the medical specialists. Not at all, say I.

One patient I will never forget was the beautiful, slim, blonde-haired 16-year-old girl who walked cheerfully into the paediatric outpatient clinic in Bristol when I was a medical student. She was dressed in horse-riding gear and was accompanied by her mother, and a group of four of us medical students were sitting in on the clinic to observe and learn. The consultant talked to her and her mother, examined her chest, briefly looked at the results of her lung function tests, and discussed antibiotics with her. He then said goodbye to them with a smile, and asked her to make an appointment in six months' time. Mother and daughter then cheerfully walked out, and, as soon as the door closed behind them, the consultant's smile disappeared. He sombrely turned to us and said that the elegant young patient we had just seen would not attend the next appointment, simply because she would be dead before then. She had cystic fibrosis, and almost no lung function left, and her next chest infection would be fatal.

Cystic fibrosis is a terrible condition. It is a congenital illness due to a faulty gene that is quite common, in that one in 25 of the population carry it. Fortunately, it is not a dominant mutation, which means that, if you simply carry the faulty gene, having inherited it from one of your parents, you do not acquire the disease. You only have cystic fibrosis if you inherit the faulty gene from both parents. When you are conceived, you get half a set of genes from your father and half from your mother, and that combination is what makes you (and makes you unique, unless there is an identical twin). When a child is born to two parents of whom just one (mother or father) is a carrier of the cystic fibrosis gene, there is no possibility of the child having cystic fibrosis. This is why:

Father's genes: N (normal) plus CF (faulty)
Mother's genes: N (normal) plus N (normal)

Mixing N-CF with N-N has these four possibilities:

N-N   N-N   CF-N   CF-N

This means that, on average, half the children produced would be carriers, but not one would have the actual disease, because you need the combination CF-CF to have cystic fibrosis.

But if both the father and the mother are carriers, the situation changes:

Father's genes: N (normal) plus CF (faulty)
Mother's genes: N (normal) plus CF (faulty)

Mixing N-CF with N-CF has these four possibilities:

N-N   N-CF   CF-N   <u>CF-CF</u>

This means that, if two carriers get together and make babies, on average, one in four will be normal, two will be carriers, and one in four will be unlucky and have the actual disease.

Cystic fibrosis affects many organs, but the most vulnerable of all are the lungs. Patients find it difficult to clear lung secretions, so that these build up and clog the airways, leading to infection after infection, each slowly but inexorably leaving some lung damage. In the 1960s, few children with cystic fibrosis made it past the age of ten. With massive effort from parents, physiotherapists, nurses, and doctors over the past few decades, survival has improved tremendously. Nowadays, cystic fibrosis patients receive regular and vigorous physiotherapy every single day, any lung infection they develop is aggressively treated, and they are kept under close review, with care given by parents, teachers, and a dedicated healthcare team in specialist clinics. With this treatment, survival is now well into the fourth decade, and many children with cystic fibrosis now can expect to live well beyond, into their 40s.

Why am I telling you about cystic fibrosis? The reason is simple. It is one of the specialties in which one would have thought that quality monitoring is impossible. The reasons, or excuses, are legion and the following have all been said by doctors specialising in this field and in other areas of medicine:

- Our specialty is nothing like cardiac surgery.
- We cannot make our patients better — it is a slowly progressive disease.
- We don't have an outcome measure. It's so easy for you cardiac surgeons: death and survival are easy to define. We have no such thing in our specialty.
- Our outcomes are so much more subtle.
- Our patients are very different from one another in age, disease severity, and how fast the disease progresses.

In fact, none of these excuses holds water. Even a clinic that provides medical care to cystic fibrosis patients can have outcome measures. All we need to do is to ask a few basic questions:

- What is the service trying to achieve?

- Is there a reliable way of measuring that achievement?
- Is there an acceptable target to aim for?

In fact, one could easily argue (and I often do) that if doctors do not know what they are trying to achieve, have no way of measuring whether it has been achieved, and no idea if the achievement is good enough, then what on Earth are they doing in medicine? They'd be better employed selling snake oil.

Let us come back to cystic fibrosis: once these three simple questions are answered, how to monitor becomes self-evident. So here goes:

What is the service trying to achieve?
We know that cystic fibrosis cannot be cured, and that the progress of the disease cannot be stopped, so the best that can hoped for is a slowing down of the inevitable deterioration. Put on the spot, doctors specialising in cystic fibrosis agree with this statement.

Is there a reliable way of measuring that achievement?
Of course there is: all cystic fibrosis patients are monitored using lung function tests (in which they blow into tubes so that the capacity and effectiveness of their lungs can be measured). These measurements are routinely taken at frequent intervals in the cystic fibrosis clinic, and they are safe and non-invasive tests.

Is there an acceptable target to aim for?
Here we need to defer to experts in the field. They have agreed that, in general, a good thing to aim for is that lung function, as measured by the tests, should not deteriorate by more than 5 per cent per year. Achieving that would count as a success of the treatment.

The above is precisely what Dr Diana Bilton, who ran the cystic fibrosis service at Papworth Hospital in the 1990s, worked out and implemented. To the best of my knowledge, the service was the first non-surgical service in the world to introduce robust, objective quality monitoring with an actual, credible, relevant, and objective performance indicator. She proved that such practice is possible outside the narrow field of heart surgery and the wider one of surgery in general.

The value of such an approach is manifold. First, it informs the doctors, nurses, and other healthcare professionals how well they are doing. Second, it allows for the detection and correction of any underperformance (if you don't even know it's broke, there is no incentive to try to fix it). Third, it allows units to compare their performance, so that those doing less well can learn from those doing better. Finally, it allows for the assessment and audit of any treatment modification or innovation. Shouldn't all doctors in all specialties be doing this?

So, where are we now?

I am a tiny, insignificant, ignorant bit of carbon.
I have one life, and it is short
And unimportant
But thanks to recent scientific advances
I get to live twice as long as my great great great great
  uncleses and auntses.
Twice as long to live this life of mine
Twice as long to love this wife of mine
Twice as many years of friends and wine
Of sharing curries and getting shitty
At good-looking hippies

With fairies on their spines
And butterflies on their titties.

These lines are by the Australian comedian and musician Tim Minchin, from his beat poem 'Storm', possibly one the most eloquent (and funniest) eulogies to science and modern medicine that I have ever heard. It is also a viciously sharp and effective attack on alternative medicine and unscientific thinking in general. It makes you both think and laugh out loud at the same time.

A long time ago, medical treatment was simple and cheap, much of it was safe, and most of it was utterly useless. Today, medical treatment is complex and expensive, some of it can sometimes be highly dangerous, but most of it is very effective. The progress made by medicine and surgery in the past few decades has been awesome in depth, range, efficacy, and complexity.

That said, much of our enviable good health and longevity derives not from high-tech medical intervention, but from basic public health measures, such as safe and nutritious food, clean water, decent sewerage, healthy living environments, mass vaccination, and not smoking. More can be ascribed to basic healthcare such as antibiotics for infections. Quite a bit of our good health, however, comes from modern, high-tech, and expensive medicine. The contribution of modern medicine to the overall health standard of the population is still relatively small when compared with more basic public health measures, but it is undoubtedly growing.

Heart surgery alone can now fix what was unfixable with operations that were unthinkable just 30 years ago. In fact, with the rare exception of heart failure, there is now a surgical solution to almost every cardiac problem, from coronary disease to leaky valves and enlarged aortas, all the way even to surgical treatment of electrical rhythm disturbances of the heart. Even heart failure may soon become a thing of the past when the artificial heart becomes reliable and inexpensive, and that surely is only a matter of technology and time. Progress in other fields of medicine has been similarly exciting, with keyhole surgery to fix many problems in the abdomen, phenomenal orthopaedic treatments to replace worn-out joints, kidney transplants for renal failure, liver transplants for hepatic failure, and eye surgery to treat cataracts and refraction abnormalities. Even the brain, that impossibly complex organ, is beginning to yield to surgical attempts to fix it. The results of cancer treatment are massively better than they were 50 years ago, and many cancers can now be looked at as a chronic disease rather than an imminent death sentence.

Chances are that you, if you live long enough, will need and benefit hugely from one or the other of these high-tech medical solutions to problems. A substantial proportion of us, if we reach a ripe old age, will have a worn aortic valve replaced, receive a pacemaker, have a coronary bypass, and so on, and that is just in my field. More will have joint replacements, prostate treatment, operations for cancer, and procedures on the arteries and veins of the body outside the heart.

In this book, I have deliberately drawn attention to the foibles of my profession. We often work with incomplete medical knowledge. We occasionally make stupid decisions. We take unnecessary risks with our patients' lives and wellbeing. The good news is, we are finally embracing the concept of 'total quality management', albeit half a century after the Japanese carmaker Toyota incorporated it into its production systems, and we are beginning to understand risk management and safety protocols two decades after civil aviation. We still have a long way to go.

Despite this, I believe that medicine has never been better

than it is today. Our treatments are mostly effective. We can make patients feel better. We can help them live longer. Our practice is largely based on evidence. Quality assurance is rapidly becoming integral to our processes. We have started to learn from crashes and near misses, improving our methods and our systems. And there is increasing transparency in our work. In every single aspect of the improvements listed above, cardiac surgery has played the lead role. For that, my colleagues and I may perhaps be forgiven the indulgence of a little pride.

Tomorrow, or sometime in the future, you or someone you love will perhaps need a heart operation. My hope is that the material in this book will help you to ask the right questions, consider the options, and reach the right decision. If you decide to go ahead and place your life in my hands, or in the hands of one of my colleagues, you can do so with confidence. Medicine has never been as good as it is now, and nowhere is that truer than in the specialty of heart surgery.

Acknowledgements

Steve Large and Steve Bolsin generously provided me with heartfelt narratives of their experience of difficult times when they must have felt most vulnerable. My daughter Leila applied her phenomenal literary skills both to the manuscript and to the proposal, without which *The Naked Surgeon* might have never seen the light. Peter Tallack of the Science Factory is an amazing agent, whose remit extends way beyond mere representation, to include perceptive insight and excellent advice, given with passion and dedication. Philip Gwyn Jones and David Golding did a superb job in editing the final manuscript. To all of them, and to my partner, Fran, for her tireless and unwavering support, thank you.

anywhere in the UK. Nobody except the surgeons did. However, what I did know was that, in Bristol, the operations were taking a long, long time. That, by itself may not have been a bad thing, but two other factors worried me even more. Firstly, the long times on the cardiac-bypass pump led to much more postoperative organ damage than in London hospitals. Secondly, the length of time the heart was starved of oxygen during the operations in Bristol was also much longer than London, and this led to severe heart damage and children dying in much greater numbers.

A few months after I had started in Bristol, an audit meeting of the paediatric cardiac surgical specialists confirmed my suspicions that the death rates in Bristol were abnormally high. The meeting was held specifically to discuss the operation of repair of ventricular septal defect (or VSD: a hole in the heart). The mortality rate for this operation at the Royal Brompton Hospital in London and around the world was very low, at around 1 per cent. Figures were presented that indicated the mortality in Bristol for this simple operation was incredibly high, as much as 30 per cent. The problem in Bristol was not that surgeons and cardiologists were unaware of the high mortality rates; the problem was that they were not prepared to do anything to get the death rates down. In those days, holding audit meetings was revolutionary, forward-thinking, and probably ahead of many other centres with better results. However, failing to act on the evidence of these audit meetings and annual reports was typical of the attitudes in Bristol.

The paediatric unit in Bristol had been under a cloud for many years. An expert paper produced for the Department of Health in 1980 had insisted that paediatric cardiac surgeons needed to do at least 50 operations each year on children less than one year of age (infants) to maintain their skills. Units doing more than 50 operations in young children had lower mortality rates than those that did fewer than 50. Bristol had never achieved that number of operations, and had not been considered in the first list of centres to be given the prestigious 'Supra-Regional Paediatric Cardiac Surgery Centre' status by the Supra-Regional Services Advisory Group (SRSAG), chaired by Dr Norman Halliday. The description by the Committee of the Bristol unit at that time was that it 'did not shine like a star' and was 'not one of the leading lights'. Bristol was designated to fail, but was added to the list of Supra-Regional centres in 1983, as an afterthought, in response to its geographical location in the west of England. There was no consideration of high mortality rates at this stage.

The city of Cardiff, in Wales, is 44 miles from Bristol. In 1986, the senior cardiologist in Cardiff, Professor Andrew Henderson, negotiated a special arrangement with the paediatric cardiac centre in Southampton (138 miles away) to assess and treat children from Cardiff and Wales. In doing so, he was replicating a deal that the paediatricians in Plymouth (120 miles from Bristol) had negotiated with Southampton (152 miles away), also in 1986, to assess and treat their children as well. Both arrangements were specifically made to ensure that children were not treated in the 'high-mortality' Bristol centre. Nobody told the parents in Plymouth, Cardiff, or Bristol. At that time, the criticisms of Bristol were so strident the Chief Medical Officer for Wales, Professor Gareth Crompton, discussed the matter with the Chief Medical Officer for England Sir Donald Acheson. Professor Crompton was advised to speak to Dr Norman Halliday.

Also in 1986, a report co-authored by Mr Terence English had confirmed that Bristol did not have the number of operations necessary to achieve low mortality rates, but Dr Halliday's SRSAG continued its designation of Bristol as a Supra-Regional centre. By 1987, the criticism was so loud that the broadcaster BBC Wales aired a scathing documentary about the survival of children from south Wales in the Bristol centre.

My problem from 1989 was that operations on tiny babies less than one month old were the highest risk in Bristol. After consulting a senior colleague, in June 1990, I decided to express my concerns, and wrote to Dr John Roylance, who was about to become the chief executive of the Bristol Royal Infirmary. The response to my letter was swift. First, a phone call from the chief executive dismissed the concerns. Second, a meeting with the chairman of the Hospital Consultants Committee concluded that I had been manipulated by a senior colleague. Later, I attended a meeting that was much more sinister. An obviously infuriated Mr Wisheart explained that writing to the chief executive was not the way to behave in cardiac surgery, and he delivered a potent threat: 'If you wish to remain in Bristol you should not disclose the results of paediatric cardiac surgery to people outside the unit ever again.' The venomous and intense manner of the delivery of the message added to its sombre content. This was reinforced at an anaesthetic audit meeting held to discuss paediatric heart surgery some weeks later. The president of the Association of Anaesthetists of Great Britain and Ireland, himself a cardiac anaesthetist, advised caution in dealing with the issue, because, as he put it, 'Steve had already put his head above the parapet and had a "pot shot" taken at him'. This was colourful language from a colourful character, but very sobering feedback for a junior anaesthetist like me who desperately wanted to do the best for his patients.

Later that year, the annual report for the Bristol unit, which was produced by the surgeons, confirmed that the mortality for 'complex' and 'moderately complex' paediatric heart surgery was twice as high as the national average. This report confirmed that the surgeons and the cardiologists themselves knew how badly they were performing. However, their combined lack of action to improve the mortality rates indicated that they had no intention of regulating their referrals or their surgery to reduce the risk of death and serious injury to the patients they served. There was no evidence they were prepared to do anything about the high death rates, and they certainly did not warn the parents of their tiny patients.

I continued to collect audit data on my patients, including the vital outcome of whether they survived the operation to leave hospital. My figures only served to increase my anxieties about the dangerous nature of the service of which I was an integral part. I was now so convinced of the deadly nature of the operations that I decided to apply for a position outside Bristol. I approached the Professor of Anaesthesia for a reference. I explained about the paediatric heart surgery results, and he confided that he had known about the long operations since his appointment to Bristol in the 1970s. His first task in Bristol had been to adjudicate a disagreement between the cardiac surgeons and the cardiac anaesthetists about how long the cardiac surgery was taking. Now he struck a deal with me; I would collect robust mortality data on all paediatric heart surgery patients, and he would provide his senior lecturer to help in the analysis of the data if my application was unsuccessful. Andy Black and I started the data collection in August 1991.

By the summer of 1992, two audits had been conducted by Professor David Hamilton with members of the Royal College of Surgeons and the Royal College of Physicians for Dr Halliday's SRSAG in the Department of Health. The audits had confirmed that Bristol had twice the mortality rate for open-heart surgery than every other centre in the UK bar one. A letter to Sir Terence English, who was the president of the Royal College of Surgeons, from Bristol anaesthetist John Zorab, had raised the problem of high mortality at the Bristol Royal Infirmary. Sir Terence had discussed the issue with Professor David Hamilton after reviewing the professor's recent report to the SRSAG. Professor Hamilton had admitted that he and his working party had paid 'insufficient attention' to the figures in Table 1 of the report. These showed Bristol had more than twice the mortality of other centres for many conditions.

Sir Terence and Professor Hamilton then agreed to take executive action on this important issue. Sir Terence informed Dr Halliday of their recommendation that the SRSAG should de-designate Bristol as a specialist paediatric cardiac surgical centre. However, Sir Keith Ross and Professor Hamilton reviewed this decision while Sir Terence was abroad, and, in consultation with the other members of the working party, Sir Keith advised Dr Halliday that Bristol should not be de-designated because of its high mortality. The reason given by Professor Hamilton in his letter to Sir Terence was that he was concerned about 'a possible specific source of "breach of confidentiality" which could arise' and 'a further feeling that the de-designation of one of the Units would probably leak out in the course of time'. The SRSAG instead decided to de-designate all centres at their July meeting. This decision cost scores of children their lives.

Still nobody thought they should warn the parents.

By late 1992, Andy Black and I had produced preliminary results that painted an alarming picture. Compared to the national-average data from several years before, there was not a single operation for which Bristol had lower death rates, and, for several operations, Bristol had much higher death rates. The argument that Andy and I developed was that Bristol should concentrate only on the operations for which there was evidence the Bristol results were similar to the 'national average', and we should only start the more dangerous operations when there was reason to believe we could do them safely. The message was not well received at any level in the organisation. With the results verified by a paediatric cardiologist, we took them to the new Bristol Professor of Cardiac Surgery, Gianni Angelini. The results were no surprise to him because the appallingly high death rates in Bristol were the 'open secret' of British cardiac surgery.

Andy's and my audit results confirmed the worst, but no one wanted to question Mr Wisheart, who by now was the senior cardiac surgeon, head of the cardiac surgery unit, chair of the hospital medical committee (representing all the hospital senior doctors), and also medical director of the entire hospital. The situation continued to deteriorate, with many more children and babies dying unnecessarily. I made plans to give up my paediatric cardiac surgery practice.

One of the cardiac procedures for which the Bristol surgeons had an exceptionally poor record was the relatively new 'arterial-switch' operation. This is an intricate, dangerous, and technically challenging operation. In babies under one month of age, the record at Bristol was an unenviable nine deaths in 13 cases. In Birmingham, which is only 90 miles away, Bill Brawn had operated on more than 200 babies for this condition, with only one death. Nevertheless, in December 1994, Bristol surgeon Janardan Dhasmana listed an 18-month-old toddler, Joshua Loveday, for an arterial-switch operation. Gianni, Andy, and I were horrified, and set about agitating the organisation for a review of this decision. I contacted Bill Brawn, the excellent surgeon in Birmingham, who had offered to retrain Janardan after his initial dismal failure at the operation. Bill's view, from what he had seen of Janardan's capability when he had visited him in Birmingham for retraining, was that he could not, and therefore should not, do the operation. However, he forbade me from communicating his opinion to Janardan, or anyone else, as this would ruin his mentoring programme for paediatric cardiac surgeons. We both agreed to contact a Department of Health official (Dr Peter Doyle) to try to get the operation stopped. Unfortunately, the surgeons remained completely unmoved, until the night before the operation, when Mr Wisheart called a meeting to discuss the operation.

Gianni and Andy were specifically excluded, but I attended. The meeting was told that Joshua's operation was necessary and urgent. The figures for the arterial-switch operation in Bristol were compared to 'national average' figures. The sub-division of the figures into small numbers made statistical comparison with the national figures meaningless, and thus the poor record was obscured. Mr Wisheart proposed that the operation should proceed. Seeing that there were no dissenters, I took a deep breath, and said 'No'.

My argument was that the record in Bristol for this operation was poor, and had not improved since Janardan had 'retrained' in Birmingham. I included the low Birmingham death rate, adding that I had been concerned enough to raise the results with the Department of Health. This horrified the consultants, who were obviously petrified of external scrutiny. I believed that Joshua should be referred to another unit, and that operating unsuccessfully on him in Bristol would have serious repercussions. Despite fierce criticism, a vote was finally taken, and I asked my single minority view to be minuted. I did not know that Peter Doyle had contacted Dr Roylance (Bristol Royal Infirmary chief executive) regularly to get the decision to operate reviewed. Peter had also insisted that Mr Wisheart arrange the last-minute meeting. What neither Peter nor Dr Roylance expected was the agreement to proceed with Joshua's operation.

And still nobody warned the parents.

That night was the worst in the whole of my medical life. Far, far worse than the exhaustion of a 'five-day continuous on-call weekend duty' was the heartache and genuine anguish of the certainty that a child's life was being placed at risk just for surgical pride. Maggie, my wife, and I discussed the options of telling Joshua's parents to take him to Birmingham, but decided that the near certainty of having our concerns dismissed by the parents and of being de-registered or 'struck off' the nursing and medical registers made the whole mission a disaster from the start. I am still haunted by the knowledge that Joshua's parents wished we had tried to tell them the truth. In another world, I would have done so. I was not brave enough then.

The switch operation proceeded the next day, 12 January 1995. I rang the operating theatre to find out how the operation had proceeded that evening. I heard from a nervous theatre sister that Joshua was still in the operating theatre after nearly 12 hours of continuous operating. I knew then that he would not survive, and, an hour later, Gianni Angelini told me that the toddler, Joshua Loveday, had just died, still on the operating table. Maggie and I cried with sorrow and anger. Our anger was directed at an institution that had cold-heartedly sacrificed a child's life for the sake of surgical pride. This was an unforgiveable act, but who would hold anyone to account?

The Department of Health decided that external investigators should review the Bristol paediatric heart surgery service. The reviewers invited by the hospital were Marc de Leval, a consultant cardiac surgeon from Great Ormond Street Hospital in London, and Dr Stewart Hunter, a paediatric cardiologist from Newcastle, who had co-authored the 1992 report for Dr Halliday's Committee that had led to Sir Terence English advising de-designation of the Bristol centre. Stewart Hunter arrived in Bristol and met paediatric cardiologists the night before the inquiry.

On the day of the inquiry, I faced a relatively hostile inquiry team to whom I presented my information in the form of annual reports, tables, sequences of operations, and graphs, all packaged in clear plastic envelopes. It was not until I was able to convince them that the information came from multiple sources, including the surgeons themselves, that I was given any credibility.

The first report produced by the 'independent reviewers' concluded that Mr Wisheart must be seen as a 'higher-risk surgeon' and should cease paediatric cardiac surgery immediately. Mr Dhasmana should retrain in the arterial-switch procedure, and could continue other paediatric cardiac surgery operations. The report was completely unacceptable to the hospital and at least one of the surgeons. When Dr Roylance returned from his holiday, it was 'rewritten'. Sadly, no one remembers by whom. This decision cost another young child, Andrew Peacock, his life. He was operated on by Mr Wisheart on 1 May, which was the same day that Ash Pawade, the new, safe paediatric cardiac surgeon started. Andrew died of brain damage a month later. His parents were never told of the findings in the first report that Mr Wisheart was 'a higher-risk surgeon'.

I do not know to this day who 'rewrote' what sections of the report. The second version claimed that the concerns of the anaesthetists had so undermined the confidence of the surgeons that they had been unable to operate successfully! In this Orwellian organisation, the source of the problem was redefined as not the surgeons, but the anaesthetists. The 'revised' report was released to the BBC in Bristol, and I believed I had a right to defend myself as one of the anaesthetists allegedly responsible for the high mortality. I was advised by senior colleagues not to attend the interview, but I felt strongly enough to complete an interview, on camera, with Matthew Hill for BBC television.

The same week a reporter from *The Daily Telegraph* newspaper contacted me to discuss some figures for death rates from cardiac surgery operations, and an article was published in the *Telegraph* the next day. My first task that morning was to explain, in person, to Dr Roylance how the highly damaging results for paediatric cardiac surgery in his hospital had been spread across the front page of an influential daily paper. It was an uncomfortable experience, but I was helped by the fact that the *Telegraph* had misspelt my name. In the end, I was accused of nothing more than naivety in handling a press inquiry, but, as I left Dr Roylance's office, he made a very curious comment. 'You know, Steve, you were right, but you were too young.' It left me puzzled and frustrated. It meant that he knew that there was a problem in paediatric cardiac surgery, that I was doing the right thing in highlighting the issue, but that he would allow the senior clinicians to hold sway over the children's best interests. I felt very strongly that it was an immoral and unacceptable attitude. However, my opinion meant very little in the Bristol management structure, and the concerted cover up continued.

Parents were still none the wiser.

As the legal cases against the Bristol Royal Infirmary mounted, investigations revealed that, in at least one case, operated on by Mr Wisheart, crucial evidence had gone missing. The ICU chart, confirming an avoidable, medical cause of permanent brain damage in a child, had disappeared shortly after Mr Wisheart had withdrawn it from the medical records department. My legal report at the time confirmed the facts.

I visited local MPs Dawn Primarolo and Jean Corston (now

Baroness Corston), and questions were asked in the House of Commons. Unfortunately, the answers remained evasive, and the true position was not disclosed. However, parents were becoming more involved and more determined to expose the truth. Michaela and Stephen Willis from North Devon, whose son Daniel had died during arterial-switch surgery by Mr Dhasmana, were pursuing answers through their member of parliament, Nick Harvey.

I applied for positions in other English hospitals, but also considered Australia. I secured a position as Director of Anaesthesia in Geelong, Australia, starting a new cardiac surgery service. I was then approached by James Garrett, an investigative journalist working in Bristol. I was now prepared to tell the whole, disgraceful story, but my fear of the medical establishment in England meant the programme was broadcast after I had left the country. 'Broken Hearts' went to air in April 1996. The next day, an article entitled 'Why Did They Allow So Many to Die?' was published in *The Times*. The author, Sir William Rees-Mogg, was from Bristol. The article was highly critical of the hospital management, naming and shaming both Mr Wisheart and Dr Roylance.

I also wrote to the General Medical Council (GMC), the official body that regulates doctors in the UK, and reported what had happened in Bristol, suggesting it might constitute 'serious professional misconduct'. I was subsequently told I was the only doctor to report the events in Bristol to the GMC, and I believe this failure remains an indelible stain on the medical profession in the UK at that time. The GMC were forced to take firm action, and recommended an inquiry. This turned out to be the longest and most expensive inquiry in their 140-year history. The inquiry confirmed that children had died in Bristol who would have survived had they received care in other centres.

The findings of the Disciplinary Committee of the GMC were announced in 1998. Chaired by Sir Donald Irvine, the Committee found that Dr Roylance, Mr Wisheart, and Mr Dhasmana were all guilty of serious professional misconduct. Dr Roylance and Mr Wisheart were 'struck off' the medical register, and Mr Dhasmana was to undergo retraining. Dr Roylance appealed the verdict and the sentence of the Committee. The Privy Council upheld both the verdict and the sentence, thereby confirming in law that medical practitioners in roles of medical management had as a primary duty the welfare of the patients in their care. Ignoring that duty could lead to erasure from the medical register.

Later in 1998, the Bristol hospital announced the results of an inquiry into the performance of adult cardiac surgery. Mr Wisheart had always claimed that the excessive examination of his paediatric cardiac surgery results was unfair, because these operations represented only a very small proportion of his total work, the rest of which was excellent. The results of this inquiry showed something very different.

For coronary artery surgery in adults, Mr Wisheart's mortality was nearly six times that of his colleagues. For other cardiac surgery, his mortality was four times higher. The conclusion was that Mr Wisheart found the delicate surgery involved in adult coronary surgery too difficult to do it well. He should probably never have started paediatric surgery, where structures are smaller, and suturing much more delicate. The figures on mortality had made this clear for many years, but no one, not even the Royal Colleges or the Department of Health, was prepared to tell him to stop the dangerous surgery. I am sure things are different now in the UK.

The response of the cardiac surgical community was unpredictably paradoxical. When the senior cardiac surgeon in Geelong returned from the European Cardiac Surgical Conference in 1998, he smiled as he told me I was 'the most hated cardiac anaesthetist in Europe'. It was an unexpected and bitter pill to swallow for saving so many lives. Articles in *The Lancet* and the *British Medical Journal* documented the appalling death rate in Bristol. From a peak of 30 per cent mortality in the early 1990s, the unit now became one of the safest in Britain, with a mortality rate falling to below 3 per cent only two years after I left.

I could live with the hate if the children survived.

In June 1998, the following Early Day Motion was passed in the House of Commons:

> That this House notes the courage of Dr Stephen Bolsin, the consultant anaesthetist who first exposed the high death rate and injury in heart operations on babies at the Bristol Royal Infirmary during the late 1980s and early 1990s; regrets that the tragedies were allowed to occur; notes that many of the improvements in the NHS emerging from these tragic events will be traced back to Dr Bolsin's decision to speak out knowing it could put his job on the line to do so; believes his behaviour sets an example to others; and commends his judgement in prioritising patient care above professional pressures to conceal bad practice.

The wider response was also constructive. The new Chief Medical Officer, Professor Liam Donaldson, and Dr Gabriel Scally, the Regional Medical Officer, who had watched the scandal develop under his nose, published an article outlining the principle of clinical governance. This became an accepted part of hospital medical practice around the world, and has probably saved hundreds of thousands, if not millions, of lives since its inception. I am immensely proud of this lasting contribution to patient safety, which can trace its roots back to the 'Bristol Cardiac Disaster'. My contribution to the medical profession was to update the attitude, current in the 1980s and 1990s, that 'your best was good enough'. The new aphorism was 'the best is good enough', and, to know that you were achieving the best, it was important to measure and compare the performance of units and, if necessary, individuals. Only then could patients have the confidence to approach specialists all over the country, knowing that their treatment would be as safe as possible.

The health secretary announced a public inquiry, chaired by Professor Ian Kennedy, into the management and care of children having heart surgery in Bristol between 1984 and 1995. They concluded that, for children less than one year old, from 1991–1995, over 35 children had died who would have survived had they been treated in other UK centres. The inquiry identified a 'club culture' in Bristol that had favoured the senior figures in the organisation and had placed 'too much power in too few hands'. The surgeons had 'lacked insight' and 'their behaviour was flawed'. Avoiding direct praise of individuals, Professor Kennedy highlighted my role in uncovering the problems in Bristol, and concluded: 'he persisted and he was right to do so'. The Kennedy inquiry produced 200 recommendations for the NHS, and the evidence and transcripts remain a monument to the children who died.

The final death toll for Bristol was 171 children who would have survived if they had been operated on in Birmingham or London. No parent was ever warned.

No one has ever tried to count the excess adult deaths.

Appendix B

A True Haunting

By Stephen Large

The referral slip was like all the rest: too little information and, what there was of it, haphazardly arranged. I knew that it would take a while to decipher. It lay among the 20 or so other referrals that also clamoured for attention on my desk, and there it was: the anticipated scrap of paper with written details of 17-year-old Jim, about whom the referring cardiologist had telephoned me a few days before. We'd talked in general terms about a young man, a huge aneurysm of the ascending aorta, poor heart function, and when was the right time to operate to replace this naturally weak and already hugely enlarged aorta with an artificial tube, so that imminent and fatal rupture could be averted.

I had been told that Jim was a young and otherwise healthy lad who had complained of recent, severe central chest pains that troubled him at unpredictable times. He was said to display all the characteristics of a condition called 'Marfan's syndrome': he was tall, slim, and 'double-jointed', in that he was much more flexible than most people. In a yoga class, that would be a good thing, but, in Marfan's syndrome, it means that the connective tissue is abnormal. This inherited weakness in connective tissue affects many parts of the body, but none more so than the root of the aorta, the origin of the largest artery in the body, and the one that every organ bar none depends on for blood supply. When that weakness is present, the aortic root begins to balloon out, so that its normal size of three centimetres or so increases. Jim's aortic root was a whopping 11 centimetres, way past the point at which rupture and death are a very real and distinct probability.

The aortic root is basically a tube, but one that contains some truly vital components. At its origin is the aortic valve, a delicate, gossamer-light three-leaflet structure that lets blood freely out of the heart into the aorta when the heart beats, but stops it from leaking back when the heart relaxes. Jim's aortic valve had been stretched so widely by the enlarged root that its leaflets had no chance of meeting in the middle to close and stop the backflow, and it was leaking freely back into the heart. This is called aortic valve regurgitation, and the heart does not like it. As far as the poor heart is concerned, it works hard to pump the blood into the aorta only to see most of it leak back and need to be pumped again. The heart can cope with this for a while, but was never designed to pump so much blood at every beat for a sustained period of time, and, when that happens, the heart enlarges with the volume overload and fails. This had already happened to Jim's heart: it was a bloated, weak, tired, and failing pump. The second important bit of 'clockwork' in the tube that is the aortic root is that the all-important left and right coronary arteries arise from that bit of aorta. These are, of course, the arteries that feed the heart muscle itself, and any operation to replace the aortic root needs to ensure that these arteries remain functional if the heart is to survive.

I telephoned the cardiologist, and we agreed that Jim should come over to my hospital as soon as possible so that he, his family, and I could review the picture together and agree to a surgical plan. We knew we had to deal with his aortic root as a matter of urgency, as it was about to 'pop'. At the back of our minds, we also knew that other bits of his aorta might also need attention in future, and a series of operations over time to replace the whole of his aorta 'piecemeal' was the likely scenario, but, for the time being, his aortic root was the problem that demanded immediate attention. The rest would wait.

He arrived on the ward, exceptionally tall as expected, and accompanied by his moderately tall parents. They settled into the ward quickly, and, between us, we decided that Jim would be well served by having his aortic root replaced with a woven artificial-tube graft, and a mechanical prosthetic valve to replace his own stretched and leaky one. We would also have to detach his coronary arteries from the diseased aortic root and re-implant them into the new artificial tube so as to maintain their ability to keep the heart alive. This was a big operation, with a lot to do: taking out the aortic root, leaving the coronary arteries, taking out the valve, implanting a new valve, implanting a new aortic root, re-attaching the coronary arteries to the new aortic root, and joining that to the (for the time being) relatively healthy remaining aorta that feeds the body. It was not an operation that could be conducted quickly, and as the heart would be starved of oxygen while all this was being done, and was already weak and failing, protecting the heart muscle from damage during that time would be crucial. We would use a cold solution of potassium to do this, and we would need a lot of the stuff, and we would also need to complete the operation in as short a time as possible to minimise the damage of oxygen starvation. Aortic root and aortic valve replacement, though unusual, was a familiar operation to me with my interest and focus on aortic surgery.

All agreed to go ahead, and, encouraged by Jim and his family, we even promised to take photographs during this somewhat exceptional operation. The day the operation was scheduled for finally came, and we had a detailed and carefully worked out operation plan.

We began by attaching Jim to the heart–lung machine, by placing a tube to collect the blue, de-oxygenated blood from the right atrium of the heart so that the blood could be oxygenated and pumped into one of Jim's arteries, so that the body remained alive while the heart is isolated. As we were expecting to cut away as much of the diseased aorta as we could, we would make the final join quite close to the part of the aorta that gives off the brain arteries. That would need stopping the circulation for a brief period, and, for the brain to survive that, it had to be cold, so, as soon as the heart–lung machine started, we began to cool Jim by cooling his blood from 37°C to 18°C. While the cooling was being performed, we clamped the aorta downstream from the heart, and stopped and cooled the heart with the potassium solution, planning to repeat the potassium cooling every 20 minutes to reduce any heart damage by oxygen starvation. We then opened the aorta, cut out Jim's aortic valve, and took out the aortic root, leaving the openings of the coronary arteries. We then replaced the valve with a large mechanical valve, and attached that in turn to the synthetic graft that would be the new 'aorta'. So far, all was going well and according to plan. The next step was the delicate procedure of re-implanting the coronary artery openings into the synthetic graft. The graft was about three centimetres in diameter, Jim's enormous aorta had been 11 centimetres, and so the coronary openings were too far to reach the new aorta. We needed 'extensions' to reach. We therefore quickly cut into Jim's leg, and took two pieces of saphenous vein, which we knew he could do without, and attached these to the openings of the two coronary arteries. With these extensions, we could reach the synthetic graft easily, and we plumbed them into the graft. Temperature had now reached 18°C, and it was safe to stop the circulation altogether to perform the final procedure of joining the new artificial 'aorta' to the stump of the old one, level with the branches that feed the brain.

This was completed without a problem. We flushed out any air from the heart and restarted the circulation by restarting the heart–lung machine. We also began to rewarm the blood to bring Jim's temperature from 18°C back to normality of 36–37°C. As we were doing this, the heart was again connected to the circulation, and the blood flowing down the coronary arteries washed out the potassium, so that the heart began to beat again. The surgically sewn joins looked free of leaks. We checked all surgical areas, and noted good, well-filled vein extensions between native coronary arteries and the new aorta. As we approached normal body temperature, we began to wean Jim from the heart–lung machine, and that is when the problems started.

Jim's heart was incapable of supporting his circulation. This was a very worrying development. Could this have been a troubled coronary artery leading to poor heart-muscle blood supply? We could not be sure, but, to be on the safe side, I quickly took more pieces of vein from the leg, and used them to bypass the two coronary arteries. To our utter dismay, it did not work: there was no improvement in heart function. We had little in the way of alternatives despite his youth. My hospital is a centre that offers heart transplantation for failing hearts, but it is impossible to obtain a heart from a donor on demand: such hearts are not there to be taken off the shelf — a brain-dead donor needs to be found, and that could take days or weeks. I asked for help from colleagues. We considered long-term support using a mechanical 'assist device' or artificial heart: there were technical reasons why this could not be done. All we had left was the hope that, by leaving Jim on the heart–lung machine for some more time, his heart might recover sufficiently to be able to take on the circulation so that he would survive. We did this, and to cut a long story short, there was absolutely no recovery. We had to face the fact that Jim was to die on the operating table … and indeed this is how Jim died.

I was overwhelmed. We had, I felt, undertaken all the manoeuvres to ensure the best preservation possible of the poorly functioning heart muscle, so why did it not work like it should at the end? 'Cheated' really summarised my feelings, and, clouded with this thought, I broke the dreadful and unexpected news to his worried parents. Perhaps the excessively prolonged operation had already seeded bad news in their minds. They appeared to accept this outcome in better fashion than I did.

Reflecting, as we all do in a keen attempt to accommodate and so come to terms with such events, I recognised the substantial risk of such an outcome using EuroSCORE. This is a tool we use to estimate the chance of death using pre-operative characteristics. Death was estimated to be likely to be the result in one in five of such operations, but the inescapable fact that led to Jim's death was that his damaged heart function had suffered further during my surgery.

Death is a most powerful and eloquent natural criticism, and yet more so when your patient dies before leaving the operating room, and so much more so when the patient is so very young. Even to this day, years later, I find myself reviewing in my mind all the steps of the operation, and especially those to do with the precautions we had taken to protect against hurting Jim's troubled heart further, only to find again and again that by any standards we'd done what appeared to be 'a good job', though the eventual outcome screamed that we had not. And so Jim's days in Papworth return to me often, haunting if you will, so that I certainly know these events will stay with me forever with little chance of my acceptance, accommodation, and reconciliation of them; a true haunting.

References

Arrowsmith, J. E., et al. 'Local Clinical Quality Monitoring for Detection of Excess Operative Deaths'. *Anaesthesia* 61 (5), 2006, pp. 423–426

Farid, S., et al. 'FIASCO II: failure to achieve a satisfactory cardiac outcome study: the elimination of system errors'. *Interactive CardioVascular and Thoracic Surgery* 17 (1), 2013, pp. 116–119

Freed, D. H., et al. 'Death in Low-risk Cardiac Surgery: the failure to achieve a satisfactory cardiac outcome (FIASCO) study'. *Interactive CardioVascular and Thoracic Surgery* 9 (4), 2009, pp. 623–625

Goldstone, A. R. et al. 'Should Surgeons Take a Break after an Intraoperative Death?: attitude survey and outcome evaluation'. *British Medical Journal* 328 (7436), 2004, pp. 379–382

Landsberger, H. A. *Hawthorne Revisited*. Cornell University Press, Ithaca, New York, 1958

Lovegrove, J., et al. 'Monitoring the Results of Cardiac Surgery by Variable Life-adjusted Display'. *The Lancet* 350 (9085), 1997, pp. 1128–1130

Nashef, S. A., et al. 'Risk Stratification for Open Heart Surgery: trial of the Parsonnet system in a British hospital'. *British Medical Journal* 305 (6861), 1992, pp. 1066–1067

Nashef, S. A., et al. 'European System for Cardiac Operative Risk Evaluation (EuroSCORE)'. *European Journal of Cardio-thoracic Surgery* 16 (1), 1999, pp. 9–13

Nashef, S. A.. 'What Is a Near Miss?' *The Lancet* 361 (9352), 2003, pp. 180–181

Nashef, S. A., et al. 'EuroSCORE II'. *European Journal of Cardio-thoracic Surgery* 41 (4), 2012, pp. 734–745.

Noorani, A., et al. 'Time until Treatment Equipoise: a new concept in surgical decision making'. *JAMA Surgery* 149 (2), 2014, pp. 109–111

Papachristophi, O. et al. 'Impact of the Anesthesiologist and Surgeon on Cardiac Surgical Outcomes'. *Journal of Cardiothoracic and Vascular Anesthesia* 28 (1), 2014, pp. 103–109

Parsonnet, V., et al. 'A Method of Uniform Stratification of Risk for Evaluating the Results of Surgery in Acquired Adult Heart Disease'. *Circulation* 79 (6 Pt 2), 1989, I pp. 3–12

Shahian, D. M., et al. 'Cardiac Surgery Report Cards: comprehensive review and statistical critique'. *The Annals of Thoracic Surgery* 72 (6), 2001, pp. 2155–2168

White, V. et al. 'The Effect of a Surgeon's Leave on Operative Outcomes'. *Bulletin of the Royal College of Surgeons of England* 89 (5), 2007, pp. 174–175

Further Reading

Better: a surgeon's notes on performance. Atul Gawande, Metropolitan Books, New York, 2007

Complications: a surgeon's notes on an imperfect science. Atul Gawande, Metropolitan Books, New York, 2002

Risk: the science and politics of fear. Dan Gardner, McClelland & Stewart, Toronto, 2008

The Report of the Public Inquiry into Children's Heart Surgery at the Bristol Royal Infirmary 1984–1995: learning from Bristol. Bristol Royal Infirmary Inquiry, Department of Health, London, 2001